Stardust Dreams

By Arthur C. Price III

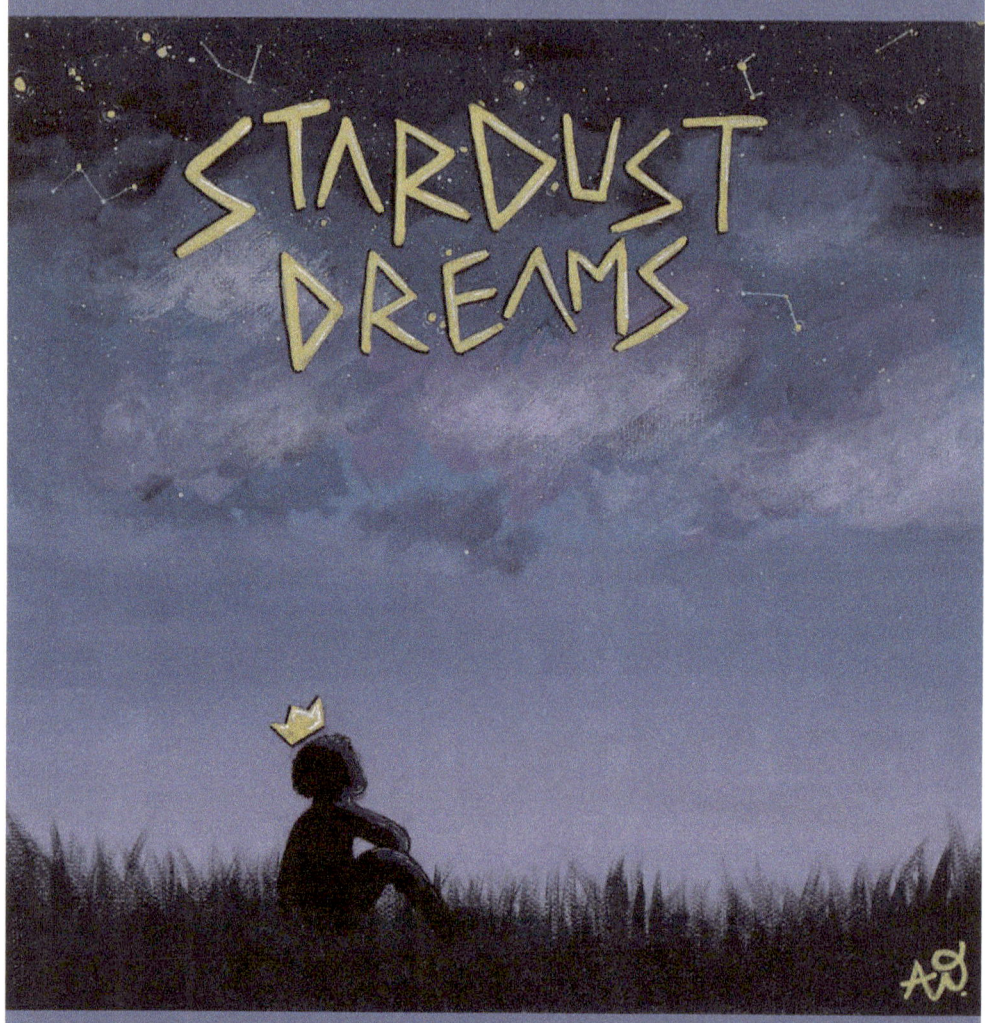

STARDUST DREAMS
Copyright Page

Copyright © 2022 Arthur C. Price III

All rights reserved. No portion of this book may be reproduced in any form without permission from the publisher, except as permitted by U.S. copyright law.

For permissions contact author: acp3@ymail.com and/or 1-225-252-6508.

STARDUST DREAMS
Disclaimer Page

All music used for this literary work is non-copyright for fair use. Credit belongs to their respective creators. I, Arthur C. Price III, do not own nor created any music used for this literary work.

STARDUST DREAMS
Dedication Page

First and foremost, this book is dedicated to the Price Family. Second, to all my friends, past and present. Third, to my coaches and teammates, past and present. Thank you to all of my loved ones to whom without, this book would have never been created.

Finally, I dedicate this book to myself, Arthur Price III.

STARDUST DREAMS

Acknowledgements

Thank you to my friend, Jared Cyprian, accepting my request to foreword this literary work. I wish you best of luck as you continue down your path. Congratulations on graduating from LSU.

"Stardust Dreams" artwork was done by Alyssa Ochoa, 2022. Please support the artist by requesting commissions and/or donating to support her art. Thank you, Alyssa, for painting a masterpiece for my book. NOTE: To support Alyssa, **please scan the QR** code at the bottom of the page. It will link directly to Alyssa's art gallery. She is open to commissions. Please take time to support her growing talents and view more of her artwork.

TABLE OF CONTENTS

FOREWORD   I-II
SOUNDTRACK   III
INTRODUCTION IV

———————————— SECTION 1: SHOOTING STAR   O

I   Leo & Lupa   2
II Galaxy-Eyes   26
III Starlit Road   48 ———— SECTION 2: DARKEST NIGHT   67

IV Black Hole   67
V   Utopia   82
VI Nightmares in Dreamland   98

———————————— SECTION 3: WISH-MAKER   113

VII Stargazer   114
VIII The Stardust King & the Castle of Dreams   126

———————————— END Painting   139-140

PHOTO GALLERY   141
ABOUT THE AUTHOR   148

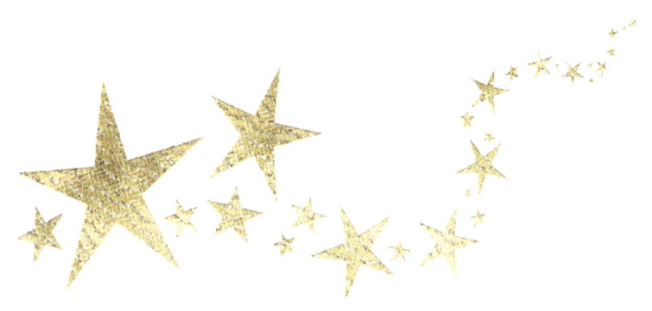

STARDUST DREAMS
Foreword

Stardust Dreams

Foreworded by Jared Cyprian

Everyone knows what it is like to dream. Dreams are the images and sensations that accompany us as we sleep. Dreams are also the thoughts and images that fill our minds as we stay awake. It is how we envision the future, hope for better days, and craft our ideal life. It is when we dream that our deepest desires come to the forefront and reflect man's intrinsic pursuit of happiness and greatness. Often in these dreams, in our visions, and in our hopes, God communicates with us our purpose and our desire for Him. And when these desires are purified, they can lead us to realize our full potential.

For that reason, our dreams are powerful and should be embraced. We can see the impact of dreams throughout human history with Martin Luther King Jr., Albert Einstein, and Mother Teresa, to name a few. Dreams are worth fighting for but they often do not come to completion without trials and tribulations. A great example of this is Joseph in the Bible. At 17, Joseph's dream was that he would rise to a position of power but it was only realized after 13 years of slavery and prison. It was through these trials that his desires were purified and he was able to grow into the man he envisioned. When speaking with his family after everything had happened to him, Joseph said "God, therefore, sent me on ahead of you to ensure for you a remnant on earth and to save your lives in an extraordinary deliverance. So it was not really you but God who had me come here; and he has made me a father to Pharaoh, lord of all his household, and ruler over the whole land of Egypt."

We all know what it is like to dream. They are not preserved for a select few but are for everyone. Another example of a great dreamer is Arthur Calvin Price III. He is a man of big dreams and someone who knows what it is like to encounter trials. But he has always been true to himself and to the God given hopes and visions, and does not let anyone or anything knock him off his course. It is not easy to stick to your dreams but in his story, Arthur shows us the power of dreams and that they are worth fighting for.

STARDUST DREAMS

Soundtrack (Interactive)

This book contains QR codes, when scanned, will play a song via YouTube link. The QR codes will be at <u>the bottom left of each chapter's illustration page.</u> The QR codes can be scanned with most phones or specific QR code scanning devices. If unable to scan the QR codes, go to the website, www.arthurpriceiii.com to find the official soundtrack. There, it will be displayed in a link, on the first page.

Track Listing

01.) Main Theme: I (Music Box)

02.) Friends Forever // Free Vibes Music

03.) Broken // Top Flow Production

04.) Agonizing Heart // Artist Unknown

05.) Way to Dream // Free Vibes Music

06.) Lamentations // Artist Unknown

07.) Titan // Scott Buckley

08.) Hopes and Dreams "Orchestrated" // Rush Garcia

09.) Main Theme: II (Piano)

STARDUST DREAMS
Introduction

Hello All,

    I hope all has been well and happiness has found you. I decided to take up authorship once more to release my second book. The overall theme of this book concerns "dreams." Dreams can be defined as many things. However, in the end, they are fantasy lands for us to escape reality.

    They are fantasy lands we desire to become a reality one day. My dream to become a king began once I wished upon a star. It is still a dream I am striving toward every day. I often look into the sky with a full heart as a reminder of the day I first began my journey. We all have hopes and dreams, so I wanted people to dive into mine. Please, enjoy this second literary work, as much time and effort have gone into it. Thank you for deciding to pick up this memoir.

    Keep your eyes in the sky and your heart in the stars. I welcome you to dive into the fantasy land that is my second book…Stardust Dreams.

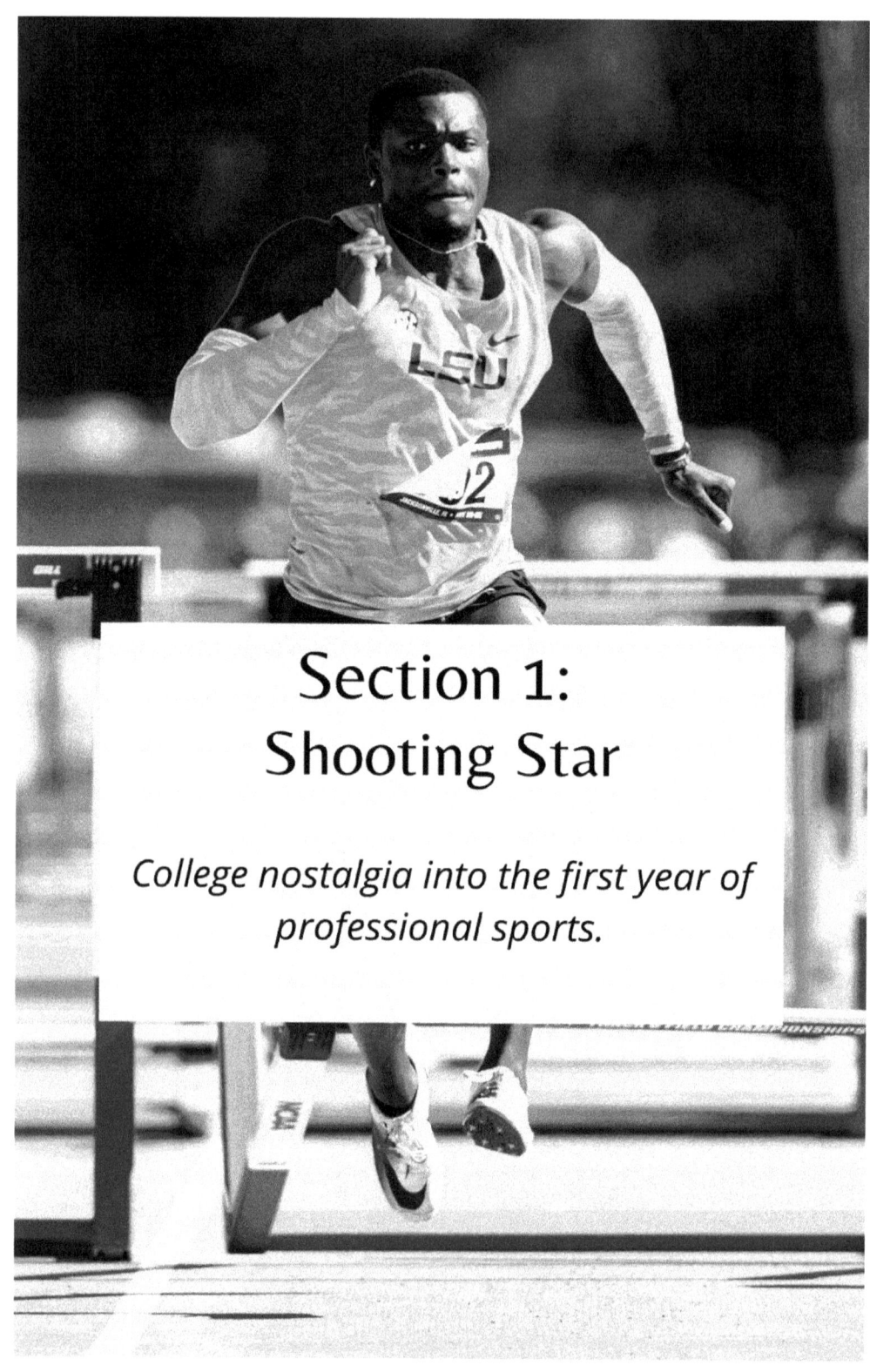

Section 1: Shooting Star

College nostalgia into the first year of professional sports.

Chapter 1: Leo and Lupa

STARDUST DREAMS

CHAPTER I: Leo & Lupa

"If we're in a simulation, I'll find you in the real world."
- Lupa

There is no perfect way to start a chapter like this. It is a chapter I never imagined I would be writing. Yet, it is a story I needed to write to close the chapter, both literally and figuratively. Life in itself is full of "hello" and "goodbyes." We don't know if it could be the last time we see a loved one. We cannot predict when we will meet someone who will change our lives. This damning realization is no need to be sad. Every heart is connected in some fashion.

Even if the connection isn't visible, the web of life connects all. I've sought this connection most of my life. Eventually, I found one person—a person who was both my opposite and equal. Even though the sun craves the light and the moon basts in the dark, both share the same sky. The same duality perfectly describes my relationship with that person--a girl. I was the proud lion, unafraid to shine my light. She was the mysterious wolf who felt solace in the darkness. This is the story of Leo and Lupa.

  Fall 2017 was the beginning of my career on the LSU track and field team. This period was one of the more challenging adjustments in my life. After receiving word of being added to the roster, I felt anxious. I knew my life was going to change, track-wise. I underestimated how much I would grow as a person. In retrospect, it was destiny for things to occur in the manner they did. I wouldn't have been reclassified as a junior if I had never taken two years off from track before 2017. If that never occurred, I wouldn't have had the chance to meet Lupa, being that she was two years under me.

  The first year on the team was a lonely one. It was hard to form bonds with most of my teammates. Simply put, we had nothing in common besides being athletes. Lupa was like me, an outsider in the group. It was something I noticed the first time hearing her speak. "I saw the new episode of Riverdale last night; it was pretty dapper," I heard across the athletic training room one day.

I turned my head to look upon a nerdy, glasses-wearing girl I hadn't noticed until then. Her demeanor was not intimidating, yet I could tell she was ambitious.

Based on how she carried herself, she desired the spotlight. However, there was another side to her I could easily see--darkness. Almost as if she wanted to bask in the light because she was too accustomed to the dark. In short, my lion-hearted nature took an interest in this new apex predator, a lone wolf.

Not knowing much about Riverdale, I responded, "yea, I love that show." My response was far from the truth as I had only seen brief clips of the show. Although it looked polarizing, I never truly invested time into it. That didn't matter to me because I just wanted to make a friend or talk to someone regarding a subject besides athletics. Unbeknownst to the time, my little white lie would start something unique. From that day forward, I befriended the same nerdy, glasses-wearing girl who I would call Lupa.

In the earlier days of our friendship, things were very surface level. Initially, we didn't spend time with each other outside of athletics. That all changed the night we decided to see Avengers: Infinity War. I was nervous because I hadn't been to the movies in years. Movie days were something my mother and I would make common.

As the years passed, those same days became a distant memory. It was a distant memory brought back by someone different, Lupa. I didn't know how to prepare for such a marvelous occasion. Perhaps that same nervousness was why I was late picking up Lupa from her apartment. As a result, we were late to the opening night screening by a few minutes. A minor mishap, yet worth every moment spent.

  The car ride to the movies consisted of the usual surface-level discussions. However, the car ride back to Lupa's apartment was more profound. For the first time in our friendship, Lupa began to open her heart. "I want to feel like someone wants to know me," she said. That same line immediately resonated with me.

  My entire life, I've felt as if I was an outsider and that nobody wanted to form a connection with me. It was eye-opening to hear something like that from Lupa. That shared feeling was our way of saying, "we want to feel important and valued." My only response to her was, "I want to get to know you," which warranted a giant smile and tight hug from her. Dropping Lupa off at her apartment that night made me feel something foreign.

  Movie nights would become somewhat traditional between Lupa and me. Whenever a new movie hit the cinema, we would be the first in the ticket lines. The entire day would be spent as a two-person party for every superhero or Disney movie premiere. Such days would later be dubbed "Geek Nights" by both of us. There was never a single dull moment during "Geek Nights."

There were constant discussions about our shared time on the following days. We would even have "insider jokes" between us, which piqued the curiosity of others. Indeed, it was a friendship I had longed for and wanted to keep. Yet, in some aspects, it still felt surface level. Although Lupa was beginning to open up more, I still felt there was a wall between us. I wanted to tear down that wall to form a closer bond. I began to contemplate why I wanted to do such or even how I would create a deepened bond. Then, the damning realization hit me – I had feelings for her.

I thought to myself, "I can't tell her; it will ruin everything." That thought was followed by "but maybe she feels the same." My mind was racing with self-created situations. My anxiety was in full swing, and I knew the best thing to do was to confront the problem. I knew being straightforward was the right thing to do, but I still was afraid. After the season had concluded, I decided to confess my feelings to Lupa during the summer of 2018. My goal was to tell Lupa in person, yet couldn't due to fear of her potential response. I don't recall the exact words, but I texted her my "crush confession."

It wasn't until a day later Lupa called me while I was driving back home from a summer class. "Arthur, I think it's best we chill out until fall training." At that moment, I was slighted but not wholly saddened. I didn't go about things properly, yet it helped me grow. With the season coming up, my mindset was to prove everyone wrong. I couldn't focus on Lupa because my dreams were more important.

During the 2018 fall training session, I was motivated yet lonely. I got into multiple fights with teammates because I wanted to send the message – I'm different now. I didn't care about what anyone thought of me. I was going to make the upcoming season my best one yet. Some days were more challenging than most because Lupa would be at practice as well. Seeing her, but knowing she wanted nothing to do with me, sucked. I would often find myself acting obnoxiously to gain her attention.

Towards the end of October, Lupa randomly contacted me. It was a brief, honest talk that led to us becoming friends once more. Naturally, I was happy to have my best friend back. However, the happiness I felt was followed by an uneasy feeling. "I can't do anything to lose her again," I thought. That singular thought was the beginning of my overall change in approach regarding our friendship. I began to tread lightly and, above all else, refused to admit my lingering romantic feelings for Lupa. I didn't want to push her away.

I figured over time, those same feelings would peter out. But unfortunately, our mended friendship only lasted a few months. In December, my emotions intensified, which led to another rift between Lupa and me. I honestly figured it was the last time we'd associate with one another. Around this same time, my mother passed away. In retrospect, I overcame a lot before the 2019 season had begun. My heart was fractured in so many places. Still, I had to endure the pain to focus on what mattered most – having a great season.

Eventually, Lupa and I mended our friendship once more in late February of the 2019 indoor track season. Although we didn't speak for two months, our friendship dynamic didn't change. The indoor campaign had just concluded. Both of us were motivated to be successful for the outdoor season. Surprisingly, there weren't any issues during the 2019 outdoor season. I genuinely believe Lupa, and I encouraged each other to be successful.

Due to our outstanding performances, we both concluded the 2019 outdoor season as All-Americans. We expected to exceed our limits next season as well. We definitely grew closer during that outdoor season. Our two previous rifts caused us to understand each other more. I am a firm believer that conflict is necessary for growth. The previous conflicts we had pushed our friendship to blossom into something extraordinary.

The summer after our fantastic 2019 track season, Lupa and I grew much closer. The summer of 2019 is something I'll never forget. Almost every other day was spent time with Lupa. There wasn't a single uneventful day between us that summer. We would often go on leisurely adventures or have movie nights at her apartment.

I began to peel the layers Lupa had previously established. As proof of her breaking down her walls, Lupa allowed me to read her diary. The act was the most powerful one yet between us. A diary is something very near and dear to its author. The words and how they are written reflect a person's emotions. Reading her diary was essentially Lupa allowing me to peer inside her heart entirely.

At that moment, my heart responded with both sympathy and empathy. Later that same day, Lupa told me something I would never forget. "If we're in a simulation, I will find you in the real world," she said. I never understood what she meant as I thought it was a reference to her favorite movie at the time. Still, for some reason, her words touched my heart. It was as if this person truly cared for me, no matter what.

Although our hearts grew closer, we were only friends. It was understood by both of us that my romantic feelings didn't have a place in our friendship. While the feelings I possessed intensified, I gained a sense of control over them. My friendship with Lupa was more important than my personal feelings. However, I unknowingly invalidated my feelings with this mindset.

In comparison, Lupa possessed the ability to express her newfound deepened feelings towards me. While these feelings may have conveyed some romantic undertones, Lupa never openly admitted anything along those lines. By her admission, she was attached to me emotionally. Being attached to someone emotionally does not equate to romantic feelings. The deep emotional bond we shared began to blur our previously established friendship line. My heart and mind were confused. The uncertainty and fear I felt were unhealthy as well.

Even though our friendship had been going strong since the summer, I needed to come clean. So, one day after track practice in November of 2019, I admitted my feelings once more to Lupa. Much to my surprise, she didn't push me away. Yet, I still pulled away from her due to my embarrassment. It was not the first rift between us. However, it was the first rift initiated by me. Ironically, a month later, Lupa and I found ourselves friends once more. However, things were different this time.

The overall dynamics of our friendship changed. In the past, Lupa held most of the power in our friendship. That all changed once I pulled away. It was apparent Lupa was acting differently, almost as a faux girlfriend. Perhaps pulling away helped her realize the latent feelings she possessed towards me.

Lupa began to display clear romantic signs such as being clingy with bits of jealousy included. There were even moments Lupa would grow angry due to slow replies via texting from me. It was apparent she didn't want to lose me again. It began to feel like she viewed me as an object for her happiness, not a person. It was a role I didn't like yet still played to appease my best friend.

I didn't know how to handle the situation. Once more, I had an internal conflict. "Do I reciprocate Lupa's energy or downplay everything" I contemplated. If I reciprocated her energy, I was at risk of misinterpreting everything. If I downplayed everything, I might miss out on leaving the friend zone. Although I possessed romantic feelings, I was comfortable just being best friends. On that same note, it was apparent we were best friends who deeply cared for one another.

I tore my hamstring in the first race of the 2020 indoor track season. I initially downplayed my injury and neglected to tell Lupa. I did so to maintain the facade of confidence. In truth, I wasn't very confident I could perform to the best of my ability while injured. Although we were friends, I admired Lupa. The admiration I held for her motivated me to be successful. However, once I injured myself and started running slower times, I felt unworthy to be around her. Not just her but everyone on the track team as well.

After the second meet of the season, I lost grip on my mental state. I felt a detachment from the real world. This feeling of detachment extended to Lupa as well. I remember walking outside late at night to clear my mind. I needed to re-gather myself and focus.

It was there I happened to walk past Lupa, being oblivious to her presence. It was very unintentional, yet Lupa took it to heart. I apologized to her the morning thereafter, but her face and demeanor were unforgiving. Lupa eventually caved in and forgave me per usual conflicts. However, I sensed a different vibe from her altogether.

Just one week later, another conflict arose between Lupa and me. At the time, I didn't think much of it. We experienced multiple friendship breakups, alongside brief periods of our egos conflicting. This time, things were very different. Lupa began to ignore me and created distance between her and myself. The week after our "cold war" conflict was my birthday.

Even my birthday didn't warrant attention from Lupa, as birthday wishes never came from her lips. Lupa was acting at a full 180 degrees from what I was used to. It was almost as if she grew to despise me. I didn't know what was happening and decided to end the standoff. I initiated contact with Lupa and planned a "sit-down" in an attempt to fix the newest rift that was forming between us. Unfortunately, I never had the chance to do so.

It was a chilly Wednesday in February of 2020. I parked my car outside of Lupa's apartment and waited for her. I was confident both of us would walk away from our talk with a better understanding. I remember the feeling of anxiety creeping through my stomach. "After this talk, we'll be okay," I thought. After about 10 minutes of patience, Lupa finally entered my car. Her demeanor was different, almost demonic-like. She carried herself as though she was another person, a stranger.

Lupa removed her phone from her pocket to set a 30-minute timer. "I'm setting this timer because I don't want to be here right now," she said. Then, Lupa began to read from her written notes a speech that changed my life. While I don't remember most of what she said, I remember how it hurt. The gist of her speech was simple: she wanted nothing to do with me, never did, and admitted to just using me for various things. She also said, "you're a jealous, clingy person who lacks independence." Every word she uttered shattered a piece of the fantasy image I had created of her in my mind. She wasn't the person I made myself believe she was.

In response to her speech, I tried pleading my case in a desperate final attempt. "No, Lupa, I can tell I hurt you, but this is a misunderstanding," I stated. "Arthur, you're being selfish right now," Lupa uttered from her mouth. Simply put, I was left speechless. I didn't know what else to do besides just ask her one final question. "What is going on right now"? Lupa's response was simple, "that is something you can figure out on your own time." Then in a blink of an eye, she was gone.

Lupa never honored the 30-minute timer, as our exchange was briefly 5 minutes. Lupa seemingly abandoned our friendship. No, she admitted we were never friends. I was left hurt, confused, and lonely. I proceeded to stare out my car window for 10 minutes. I told myself, "She'll come back; maybe she needs to blow off some steam." After those 10 minutes had passed, I knew it was indeed over this time.

I drove home and went to sleep, praying our friendship would be mended. I didn't understand why she seemed different. I couldn't fathom how all the good times we shared would equate to her going about things in such a manner. The things she said confused me. She claimed I was clingy yet would be angry if I didn't give her attention. She claimed we were never friends, yet once drew our names in a heart. I was utterly confused and mentally defeated.

Due to COVID-19, the 2020 track season was cut short. As a result, I was given another year of eligibility for collegiate athletics. I returned to LSU for one final season of collegiate athletics. I wasn't comfortable in the athletic environment because I would constantly try to avoid Lupa. I neglected to go to the training room for treatment because I didn't want to cross paths with her.

I felt uncomfortable anxiety daily at practice. I was forced to be around someone that hurt me. It was apparent Lupa was adamant about having distance between us.

Her aura was different, almost narcissistic. Even though we never spoke the entire 2021 season, there were moments I overheard her throwing slight insults in my direction. Overall, she was disrespectful and reclusive the final year we "shared" together. Even once in the weight room, she interrupted my workout for seemingly no reason. In retrospect, I deduce this was her way of trying to elicit a response from me. Maybe she wanted to talk to me but didn't know how to other than to make me angry. Perhaps, I allowed myself to remain angry out of spite. It was unhealthy, and I knew that I needed to move on to grow as a person.

With the 2021 postseason on the horizon, I needed to refocus on track. I had to remove the strife that resided within my heart. In short, I needed closure on my terms. I decided to write a letter to Lupa in an attempt for such closure. Lupa was also graduating at the time. So, I decided to include two of her favorite pieces of chocolate with the letter in a sealed envelope.

    I could not give Lupa the gift myself due to my rollercoaster of emotions. Instead, I decided to give the envelope (with the contents mentioned earlier) to a mutual friend hoping Lupa would receive it indirectly. Although I received confirmation that she accepted my gift, I am unsure if Lupa ever read my letter. I never investigated the matter further because I knew I did the right thing. Though I have a slight hunch Lupa did read the letter.

    There was a small instance at Regionals where I allowed her to use my track blocks. After taking the blocks, she took a few steps back and thanked me. The tone behind her voice was that of a thankful long-lost friend. The conclusion of

Regionals was the end of my final collegiate track season in 2021. After that, I never heard from nor saw Lupa again.

    I wanted to include this chapter to close Leo and Lupa's story. The thing is, people, come into our lives for a reason. Nobody is meant to stay in our lives forever. However, the people we have the opportunity to meet will forever impact us. Although Lupa and I weren't destined to remain friends, I learned a lot from her.

    There were various aspects of our interactions that brought out our latent talents. Lupa taught me so many things, even after our friendship ended. Instead of making myself the victim, I decided to move forward with a smile. God granted me the opportunity to meet a unique person. To this day, I am thankful for that.

    In truth, the Lupa I knew doesn't exist anymore. The version of Arthur that Lupa knew doesn't exist anymore either. The people that knew each other changed for the better. Our roads diverged when Lupa walked out of my car that fateful day in 2020. Sometimes, I do find myself thinking of Lupa. However, there's no use in mentally staying in the past. The past reminds us how far we have come.

Time doesn't stop for lost love. I pray for Lupa's success every day. If our roads cross again, I am sure we will be friends again. While Lupa still has a place in my heart, her place in my life is something I cannot control. Therefore, I have no regrets when from our friendship. Although, admittedly, there were times I did fall short.

To this day, I'm still unsure why Lupa pushed me away. Though her existence in my life was only a fraction of my lifespan, it was memorable. The shared time between us often feels like a far-off dream. Lupa was truly the person of my dreams who never existed. The memory I have of Lupa is the memory I have of nobody. Ever since she left my life, It is almost as if she never existed.

STARDUST DREAMS

There was never a perfect way to write this chapter, as I said before. Lupa was but a vapor in my life. There were so many things I could have included but chose not to. In truth, I could have written an entire book about my interactions with Lupa. However, condensing everything into one chapter will never do the story its justice.

Lupa was one of the most special people I had the chance to meet. She wasn't just my best friend. Lupa was someone I considered to be my other half. Losing her was almost like losing a part of myself. I will never meet another "Lupa" in my life, only people who have similar aspects to her. That alone makes Lupa a particular person, deserving of a place in my heart and book.

To the reader, I impose this final message. In this life, we must accept the things we cannot change, change the things we can, and have the wisdom to know the difference. Yes, the past hurts, but we can either run from it or learn from it. Matters of the heart are not easy, but we must never forget that they are still with us. In this life, nobody is ever truly gone.

To Lupa, if you ever manage to read this book, know I appreciate you. I will always cherish the time we shared. If we are meant to find each other once more, let it be not as enemies but as old friends. I am uncertain if that day will arrive, yet I am confident in one thing. I am confident in the people we will both become. And so, just as you once told me, I will say to you. "If we are in a simulation, I will find you in the real world."

I have accepted the past for what it is. I have changed my focus. My dream is still alive and well, just as I am. Now, I walk tall into the next chapter with my heart full of newfound wisdom. Perhaps the prideful Lion might see the lone Wolf again – one day, someday. See you, wolf girl.

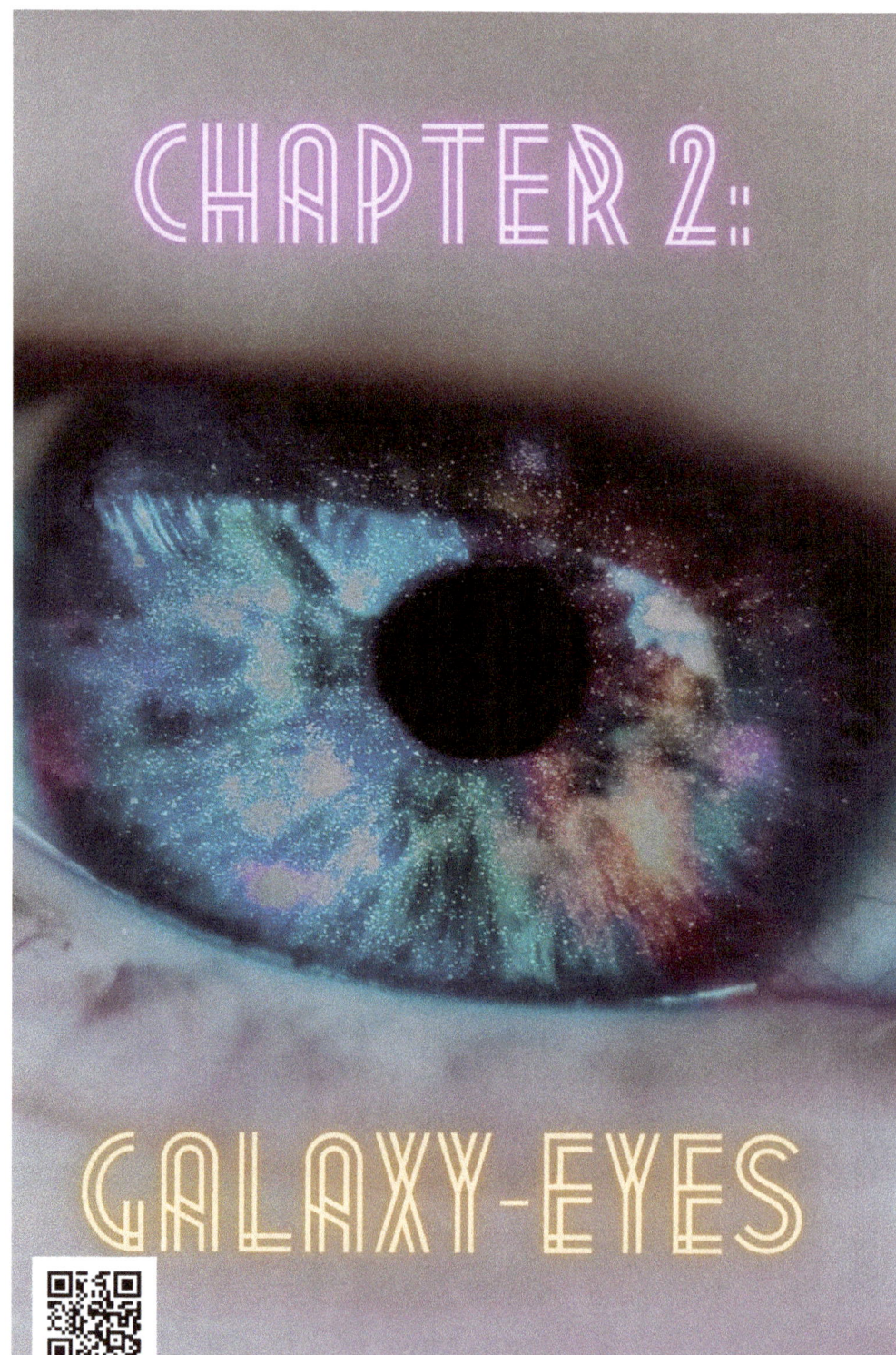

CHAPTER II: Galaxy-Eyes

"Part of the journey is the end."
            - Robert Downey Jr.

Just like the previous chapter, this following one is something I have re-written countless times. There is no perfect way to write a chapter like this. I could write an entire book on my experiences at LSU. Although Louisiana State University was only a fraction of my life, it was a significant phase. As a child, I would have never imagined my experiences in college. A dream that a bright-eyed child first dreamed. Experienced by the narrowed-eyed young man. Now re-told by the dim-eyed yet thankful adult.

Growing up, the only thing most people were concerned about in the Fall was football, mainly LSU football. Every young man's dream at the time seemed to be the same: to play football at LSU. Eventually, I became one of those same young men. But unfortunately, I wanted to play football at LSU for seemingly all the wrong reasons. I wanted to perform in front of a big crowd, get the girls, have a storied career, then ride off into the sunset. But, funnily enough, I did have that same experience, just with track and field.

To start things off, I love Louisiana State University. Attending LSU was indeed a dream come true. Only a few people can become D-1 college athletes. Even fewer are successful at the D-1 level. I was fortunate enough to be one of those select few. Initially, I didn't have the same level of appreciation I do now for the university. In truth, I hated my last year at LSU with a burning passion. While it was a very forgettable, anticlimactic year, it is one I look back on with appreciation.

To summarize my final season at LSU, it wasn't the ending I imagined. To be blunt, my last year at LSU was miserable in various ways. Once the 2019 track season ended, I figured the gained momentum would lead to "legendary" status. After all, I had just become an all-American. I felt like nothing could stop me. Ironically, the only person who stopped me was myself.

I wasn't mentally stable in the final years of my LSU career. My mental apparatus was very fragile due to a multitude of hardships. These hardships included my mother's death, falling at NCAA Nationals, my hamstring injury, and losing the bond I had with Lupa. For the first time in my life, I felt empty in seemingly every way possible. During that period, failure's aura could be felt around every corner.

In the earliest parts of Fall track training in 2021, I began experiencing crippling anxiety. Although I have struggled with anxiety for most of my life, the pressure I felt then was much different. Aside from being draining, it was also sickening, almost to needing to vomit before practices. Some of this anxiety was caused by being around Lupa, as we shared the same environment. Going into that year, I expected us not to be around each other that often.

However, life had a different plan regarding the situation. My maturation allowed me to realize that Lupa's presence affected me early on. Yet, I wasn't mature enough to prevent myself from being unbothered. It was my last season ever in an LSU jersey, so I needed to focus. I had big dreams both on and off the track. I refused to allow anything to get in the way of that.

As a result, I decided to reach out to a sports psychologist a few weeks after realizing how crippling my anxiety was. The decision to seek out mental help saved my life in many ways. Talking to my psychologist allowed me to release the pent-up strife I experienced. At first, I was timid to do so, but my emotions began to pour out more freely and smoothly over time. Initially, therapy didn't quell my anxious feelings. Yet, those same feelings became bearable as time progressed.

There were other hardships I had to overcome during that Fall training period. I began to feel "blacklisted" amongst everyone. I didn't get along with a good portion of my teammates. There were even instances Lupa threw insults behind my back. It felt like I was diving into toxic waste every time I had to be around the team, including Lupa. Every day felt like a mental battle, one I was losing. If it wasn't for the therapy sessions I attended, I am sure I would have had a total mental breakdown. My mental state was fragile, then suddenly, one day, it all changed.

As many readers know, I love superheroes. My passion for geek-related things usually pushes me toward buying anything superhero-related. Hence, why I decided to purchase a newly released video game at that time, Spiderman: Miles Morales, for the PS4. November 12, 2020, was a day I set aside solely to binge play my new video game purchase. However, there were other motivations to purchase that video game as well.

One reason is Miles Morales, and I share one visual trait, our blackness. I could easily relate to Miles Morales being a young black male. Another reason was I wanted to fully immerse myself in a world aside from the one I experienced daily. Playing through that video game was quite the experience. There was a central lesson told by the story narrative as well.

The life-changing lesson I learned was to "let her go." Even though we shared the same daily environment, I had to let go of Lupa. Lupa's presence caused me to become so distracted that I began to lose my ambition. To focus on what I desired most, I had to let her go to win an individual championship. I couldn't allow one person to have dominion over my soul. Almost two weeks later, I came across a forgotten prayer from my childhood, the prayer of serenity. The prayer goes as follows:

"God, grant me the serenity to accept the things I cannot change, the courage to change the things I can, and the wisdom to know the difference."

Even while writing this book, I often recited the prayer of serenity. The prayer itself is essentially surrendering to outside forces. I understand and respect the fact that not all people are religious. However, the message of letting go is still one most people can still take wisdom from. The only thing we can control in this life is the inner forces, not the outward ones.

I couldn't change my dynamic with Lupa, but I could change my mindset regarding it. And so, I did just that during that time frame in November. Quite symbolic of such a change on my part as November is the last month of Fall. With the arrival of December came cold, blistering weather, in contrast to the warmth of autumn. However, I was re-focused on my goals compared to the previous weather season.

Although I was able to have one final collegiate year, it was reserved solely for outdoor track. I could not compete as an unattached athlete in any indoor track meets at LSU. This was due to questionable SEC rules at the time preventing seniors with only outdoor eligibility from competing at indoor college track meets. So, the next best option was to run against professionals in the American Track League. I wasn't the only collegian to do so for extra races under my belt during this time.

However, the initial environment was slightly different. Immediately, I sensed an overwhelming aura of confidence and egocentrism. It was almost intimidating because I didn't feel as though I belonged. I was still coming off a very emotionally depleting part of my life. In truth, I mentally was not ready to compete alongside the professionals.

Still, it was the only way to get some races in before my final outdoor season started. In reality, it properly damaged my confidence in some regard as well. I was off schedule practice-wise as well. For the two professional meets I competed in, I had to travel to Arkansas on a Saturday and compete on Sunday. Then, return to practice again on Monday as a collegian.

The dysfunctional nature of that 2021 indoor campaign took a huge physical toll on me. I didn't have time to rest between trips, races, and practice. All of which led to my hamstring beginning to ache again. Just the previous season, I suffered a minor tear. Now, it was apparent my injury was returning.

Unfortunately, I had the misguidedness of trying to endure the returning pain. I refused to let the pain ruin my last season. I had to give it my absolute all, and whatever may come, endure it. Yes, it was a very dangerous, self-destructing mindset, but one my younger counterpart heavily embraced. It was a mindset I took into full belief going into the outdoor season, which slowly crept unexpectedly, like a stalker in the night.

STARDUST DREAMS

The first meet of my "finale tour" was ironically back where it all began, Louisiana-Lafayette. Almost poetic in fashion as my collegiate career began in Ragin Cajun red. Now, it was ending in LSU purple and gold. While I did win the race, it wasn't to my liking. My rhythm was entirely off. Also, my hamstring began tightening up mid-race, perhaps due to the cold environment. I tried to dismiss the entire experience beforehand because I knew next week was more important. Next week was the prestigious "Texas Relays" in Austin, Texas.

Texas Relays has always been my favorite meet to participate in. After all, it was the first race I cemented myself into the track world with my breakout performance in 2019. However, it was 2021, and my breakout performance was a thing of the past. Nonetheless, I felt confident because there were quite a few similarities between the 2019 season and the current 2021 season. My first race in 2019, which was also in Lafayette, was terrible for starters. Yet, the next week, I ran the race of my life.

Therefore, my goal for Texas Relays this time around was to replicate that 2019 season to improve my confidence.

While I did improve at Texas Relays, it wasn't good enough to make the final. I had to leave a day earlier, which was an embarrassment as I was the only sprinter to do so. During the entire drive back to Baton Rouge, I remember thinking, "I need to get it all out." As soon as we returned home, I went out to the track by myself and just hurdled for 2 hours. I needed to get the frustration out, fix my problems, whatever you have. I was still experiencing pain in my hamstring, but my anger and frustration provided a novocaine-like effect. My emotional displeasure was so great it outweighed my physical pain. I reached a complete state of total disregard for my body.

The week after Texas Relays came with various rollercoaster moments. I began doubting myself, even more, questioning if my lackluster performances were a result of my age. After all, I was a 25-year-old, 7th-year senior. People would often make jokes, which made me feel older. Perhaps, I started becoming what people jokingly viewed me as, expired. I even began arguing with my coaches, which I've never done before.

Even if I disagreed with my coach(es), I never expressed my displeasure around everyone. Most of these disputes were regarding practice strategies. A large part of my success in 2019 resulted from "practicing how I would perform." Yet many of these strategies I tried to implement once again were shut down by the people around me. It felt like my progression wasn't important because I wasn't running fast.

I began feeling embarrassed and just wanted to quit. I almost left track entirely that week. If it weren't for a last-minute phone call to a friend, I would have walked away from track and field that week. Instead, at the convincing of my friend, I decided to endure everything for at least one final week. After all, I had to race in Alabama that

Saturday. I couldn't afford to be in the wrong mindset.

The Alabama meet was a much-needed improvement for my psyche. I ran a season's best, finally recording a race under 14 seconds. It was not my personal best, yet it indicated I needed more confidence and volume. I was confident I could perform even better now. On the bus ride back to Baton Rouge, I remember thinking, "this is the turning point." I was ready and confident I could turn the entire thing around.

The following races after the Alabama meet were once again lackluster. My confidence was slipping once more. I started becoming frustrated again, distrusting my coaches and arguing with teammates once more. Worse of all, I started feeling anxious around Lupa again. I just didn't want to be around the environment anymore. It felt as if I didn't belong in the environment anymore. I was the oldest person on the team, nor was I viewed as a "superstar" anymore. This was evident, even in the media.

I have the utmost love and respect for every media person. Some of my best friends are sports reporters. The hard work media people do is often overlooked for numerous reasons. They're passionate about what they do as it is a very labor-intensive job. Having a great relationship with the media is something I view as important, especially as a young athlete. However, it hurt when I wasn't interviewed for a mini "homegrown athlete" series.

The sports media team interviewed every athlete raised in the Baton Rouge area. Except for me, every athlete who fitted the "homegrown" category was interviewed. Since I attended Catholic High School, I should have been interviewed since the high school is about 10 minutes down the road. I'm not telling this story to criticize anyone, but I remember the emotional pain. There were even moments when photographers wouldn't even snap pictures of me.

Perhaps it was all a self-inflicted wound towards my ego. Or rather, maybe I was slighted because I falsely associated success with attention from others. In either scenario, I was wrong to even dwell upon it. However, the "hard to swallow" truth was that the LSU program didn't view me as a star anymore. Shortly after that, I realized it was time to leave LSU.

My realization caused me to put things in the past once more. I had to put the media stuff behind me to focus on the postseason. In the postseason, anything can happen, good and bad. I was looking to retake my honor and pride back. The disrespect felt before the postseason was used as a motivator.

I wanted to slight the same people who slighted me by being successful. I was determined, comfortable, and re-grounded. In addition, I was also feeling much healthier in time for the postseason. My flexibility started to return, and my hamstring issues were beginning to resolve themselves. Things were beginning to brighten up as the first meet of the postseason arrived – The 2021 SEC Outdoor Track and Field Championships.

Admittedly, my performance at SEC's that year was not the best nor the worst. I ended up placing 8th, which was a first-time occurrence for me. Until then, I might have been the only national All-American not to make an SEC final. I took it as a positive sign, nonetheless. It seemed as though the tides of fate were beginning to blow in a different direction. My goal was to win an individual championship, yet I knew it wouldn't have "SEC" next to it. I didn't care, as the bigger goal was still alive and ahead of me. I took a moment into what unknowingly would be my last collegiate race – Eastern Regionals in Jacksonville, Florida.

The stage was set for my last dance. The last chance to become an NCAA champion was right before me. "It took three years of disappointment and learning, but I'm here to win," I thought, reassuring myself. In my first year, I didn't make it past the top 24. In my second year, I made it to

Nationals but fell in the prelims. Finally, in my third year, I looked to win the entire thing. The first task was getting through Regionals. I had the "veteran" experience, so focusing on each race was second nature.

The night before my first race of Regionals, I couldn't sleep. I was fearful of the worst-case scenario – falling short. Yet, ironically, I ran the best race of my season until that point the previous day. "This is easy," I thought to myself. Yet, deep down, something told me this was it. I didn't want to believe it and even asked people for advice. It was almost as if God told me, "Arthur, you had an amazing run, but this is where it ends."

The night before my final collegiate race, I went for a walk. I had to process my vast array of feelings. I was confident, yet afraid, certain, yet uncertain, planning for next week, either training for nationals or being at home. Everything was a contrast to each other. I was just ready to accept my fate. I just needed an answer.

And an answer is what I certainly did receive. I was in lane 6, twitchy and prematurely flexing my muscles. I was not calm; rather, I was on the edge of complete insanity. The gun fired off, and suddenly, my body moved on its own. This was it, clear ten hurdles, run fast, make nationals. Each step I took to the first hurdle felt like I was running in slow motion. I counted every single step coming out of the blocks in succession. "1, 2, 3, 4, 5, 6, 7, 8,...Hurdle". I was out like a lightning bolt.

Maybe, that bolt of lightning was too intense. I proceeded to hit the first hurdle with my lead leg foot. I felt my momentum slow a tad, but nothing I couldn't make up for during the race. "BOOM," I destroyed hurdle 2. "BANG," I obliterated hurdle 3, and so forth. I started in the first place; at hurdle 5, I was dead last, and coming off the final barrier, I managed to place 5th. While the placing mattered, the time did as well. If I managed to run faster than 5th place in the other heats, I was in a high position to make nationals.

STARDUST DREAMS

Spoiler alert, I didn't. I can't remember what I ended up placing, nor did it matter. My LSU career was over, but I didn't feel sadness for some odd reason. I walked back to our team area to coaches and teammates trying to console me with hugs and words. Their efforts, while appreciated, weren't needed as I wasn't distraught. In retrospect, maybe I was still processing everything. After all, my three years of hard work seemingly concluded in 13.81 seconds exactly.

Internally, I was happy, perhaps inappropriately. I knew this was where my LSU journey ended, and it was one I was delighted with. I started out begging for a chance and made the most of the opportunity. I became an All-American, achieved Top-10 marks in school history, and overcame adversity. I didn't have a "Joe Burrow" career, but I had an "Arthur Price III" career.

Our team went on to win the 2021 NCAA National Track and Field Championship. Even though I didn't make nationals, I was still selected to receive a ring. Admittedly, I wasn't going to accept it. I didn't feel deserving of something like a championship ring. However, after much convincing from friends, family, etc., I eventually did decide to receive the championship ring.

I'm happy I did just that; rather, I'm appreciative. To this day, I view the ring as a symbol for all the beautiful memories I made throughout my time at LSU. I am not a materialistic individual, yet it is perhaps one of my more prized possessions. One, I happily have insight every single day.

I know over time, other people will forget my career at LSU. This is simply the occurrence of most sports careers as a whole. There will always be new blooming flowers that garner more attention. It doesn't matter to me at all. I know my Top-10 times will belong to some new talent in the future. I know my All-American status doesn't determine my future success. Most of all, I know the experiences I had are now in the past. Through it all, I will cherish everything my entire life.

My time at LSU was truly a blessed six-year experience. I struggled to get through long classes and cram information for STEM courses. Walking through the quad and feeling the fall breeze hit me was a relaxing feeling. The countless relationships I made extended through my career. Going to football games and getting down on the dance floor at Tigerland. Traveling to track meets and watching movies with Lupa during flight delays.

I never expected to have so many memories in one place. There's way too much to ever condense into one single chapter. But it does beg the question, would I do it all over again? So I'll answer that question with another question. Does Mike the Tiger have a tail? Alright then, Geaux Tigers!

CHAPTER 3:

Starlit Road

CHAPTER III: Starlit Road

"If you focus on what you left behind, you will never see what lies ahead."
- Gusteau, Ratatouille

The final season of college athletics didn't go according to plan. Nonetheless, I still was determined to take the next step toward becoming a professional athlete. Competing on a large stage against quality competition was necessary to accomplish this goal. This is a stage track athletes must go through to reach their long-sought goals. It is a stage only suited for the best athletes in the world, with the chance of making history. I am, of course, referring to the Olympic Trials.

A few weeks after the conclusion of the NCAA Championships, I accepted my invitation to compete in the 2021 Olympic Trials in Eugene, Oregon. My personal best from the 2019 season was good enough to be a participant in the Trials. It was an opportunity I never imagined being blessed with. However, that same opportunity did not lack its difficulties. For starters, It was unknown how I would get to Oregon for my race. I was still in the process of contemplating my next move, life-wise. I did not have the money nor a job to make money to pay my trip expenses.

With the assistance of others donating to my cause, I was able to book a plane ticket and hotel room for my trip to Oregon. I was determined to make it there, and I did. No, I did not have a great final season. But, who's to say, I wouldn't go out there and make an Olympic Team. Anything and everything can occur, especially on bigger stages. But unfortunately, I didn't have that mindset during the training process for trials. I only wanted to compete and get a few more races under my belt.

In retrospect, that was the wrong mindset to have. It was a mindset of mediocrity I adopted from the limitations others had put on me. I wasn't determined enough to become an Olympian due to self-inflicted limits. Those limitations were a result of my lackluster performances during the season. The opinions of others became the opinions of myself. I didn't think I was good enough to be an Olympian, nor did others.

Once I arrived in Oregon, the LSU track family greeted me with open arms. I was able to practice with the team, get treated by the trainers once more, etc. It was lovely to suit up in LSU gear again while being around the same people I've come to know so well. The doubts previously had were removed once I felt the support from others. Everyone made me feel like it was the family I had become a part of.

On the day of the competition, I was strangely calm. The temperature was blazing, but I was unfazed. "I've done this before," I thought. There was no need to be nervous because it was a lifetime experience, no matter what happened. Immediately once I reached the stadium, my mindset was deadlocked on the race. The Headphones were on, the music loud, and I was positioned in a random corner, drinking any fluids I could get my hands on.

It wasn't long until I heard my name called for treatment. At LSU, it is commonplace for track athletes to get treatment before a competition. It is almost a tradition many LSU athletes, former and current, still hold to. Getting treatment before a race is a physical and mental preparation. It has become a vital regime for me, competing.

Sadly, the importance was not mutually shared. I only received about 15 seconds of treatment. The trainer working on me chose to leave to go into the stadium to wrap someone's ankle. It was not an emergency, yet the other person was more important than me in the trainer's mind. I was confused because there were already trainers in the stadium who were very experienced with wrapping ankles. Yet, the trainer working on me made the free-will decision to leave me high and dry.

It was almost the cherry on top of my final season in purple and gold. Frustrated yet focused on the race, I didn't let it get to me. However, telling the story to others made me realize how frustrated I should have been. People were more frustrated with the situation than I was. The collected opinion from most people is the trainer who essentially abandoned me was wrong.

I agree because the entire debacle was frustrating. However, I am not one to criticize. I don't attribute not receiving treatment before my race to running slow. I chose not to blame others for any result I may have, competition-wise. Even though I didn't make it past the first round, I was still blessed to have the experience.

In short, it was all a learning experience. The plan is to attend the Olympic trials once more in the future. I plan to be more prepared and motivated in that unforeseen future. Once I returned home from the Trials, I knew it was time to take the next step in my future. I needed to be serious and determined.

I needed to be frustrated at how my last collegiate season went. The frustration needed to be a motivator toward success. But, first, I needed to leave the past behind. I needed to leave LSU behind. It was something I was very ready to do. Yet, I was unsure of how to initiate the process of "removing the shackles."

Although I attended LSU for six long years, the school was a large part of my life for more than a decade. As a child, I dreamt of going to LSU and becoming an athlete. This also meant reaping the benefits of being an athlete, including fame. Almost every phase of my life beforehand felt like a stepping stone to LSU. Once I reached that pedestal, there were more steps I had to walk toward the top.

Once I reached the top, it became apparent LSU wasn't in front anymore. Instead, it was behind me, shrouded in darkness. I knew the time to move on and let it go had arrived. But, I was afraid to leave something like that behind. Graciously, I knew the memories made and the people I met would be alongside every step forward.

It wasn't long until I started giving away a good bit of my LSU gear during the summer of 2021. Being an LSU athlete, there is almost way too much gear received. Most of the gear I gave away was either never or seldomly worn. During my time at LSU, excluding my first year on the team, I barely wore anything with purple and gold on it. Maybe it was a personality statement or just tired of wearing the same color scheme. No matter the case, I didn't wear anything "LSU" related unless I had to. There were the rare occasions I would wear LSU gear willingly. Yet for some reason that time, on that fateful day, things changed.

On a random day in the summer of 2021, I was doing a workout in the weight room. Ironically, I had chosen to wear LSU gear due to not having other workout clothes readily available. I looked in the mirrors stationed in the weight room and felt anxiety. I had been involved with LSU in some capacity for six whole years. Yet, for some odd reason, wearing LSU clothes again as a post-collegian made me feel off. The feeling of being stuck rushed throughout my body. Some of my friends signed shoe deals and moved on with their post-college lives.

In short, they grew out of the little nest they called "college." For some reason, I didn't feel any growth because I didn't know my next move. The past six years were already planned out for me. Now, It was time for me to start living life and become an adult. I needed to stop wearing LSU gear to leave my college days in the past once and for all. I desired to feel any form of progression. I needed to feel as though the newest chapter of my life was about to begin.

I left the weight room that day without finishing the workout. The realization I had prompted me to make an immediate change. I needed to break away from the past years. I needed to do so in a manner that made me feel progression. Eventually, the motivation drove me to form a "mini" partnership with Adidas as a brand affiliate.

The collaboration allowed me to get various pieces of Adidas gear at a very affordable price.

Adidas is a brand I hope to sign a deal with in the future. However, ridding myself of the Nike logo I donned for years as an LSU athlete was mentally satisfying. The next step was figuring out how to spend all my free time. I finished with an undergrad in 2019 and tried my hand at Graduate school in my final two years of college athletics. No college athletics or academic curriculum meant I had time to do something to progress as a capable adult.

I still wanted to run track. There was a voice in my ear telling me to "continue." It was perhaps the one certainty at that time. However, I needed to find a job to support myself as an adult. I wanted a job that would benefit me in the future in some fashion as well. I did not want a job working in retail or a restaurant. I graduated college with a major in psychology and a minor in chemistry. I needed a STEM-related job to help gain experience for my future career(s), post-professional sports.

During that summer, I applied to a psychology clinic yet was turned away due to being a "male." It was odd to hear the apparent job discrimination, but it gave me experience for the real world. It was a job I had already planned to be hired for. It was also a job I desperately wanted and needed. Simply put, I was broke and needed some form of income. As a grown man, I needed a way to be financially settled. "Perhaps if I was more qualified, I could get an even better job in the future," I contemplated. Then, I decided to go back to school as a graduate student.

However, I made certain LSU was not a candidate for that. I was tired of LSU due to all the years spent there. Going to graduate school wouldn't just provide me with money. It would allow me to further my education to have better job options. A master's degree would hold more weight than a "lowly" bachelor's degree. At least, that's what employers may think.

Whichever graduate school I chose, there was a possibility I would move to that area, even if it meant across state borders. I was wholeheartedly ready to leave Louisiana and venture into the world. I sent my application to multiple schools. These were schools in states I envisioned living in. It came down to three different schools, Arizona State, NC-State, and Syracuse.

Moving to another state meant I would need a new coach. NC-State's hurdle coach is the great Allen Johnson. Learning from him would've been a great experience. However, the hurdle coach at Syracuse was also proven to be qualified as he helped mold various talents, such as Jarret Eaton. I chose Arizona State due to Coach Johnson never replying to my email and the hurdle coach at Syracuse not having the space to train me.

In the end, Arizona State was a perfect choice for graduate school. Primarily due to being able to attend graduate school remotely. To add, I even managed to get hired for a 20-hour remote position as a teacher's assistant (TA) for online classes at ASU. This arrangement allowed me to stay in Louisiana and train with my college coach Dennis Shaver. It also gave me a chance to manage my finances better and have a stable income.

Even as I write this, my financial goal is to always have at least $1,000 in my bank account. Above all, it made me feel like I grew as an adult by focusing on the future and not being "one-dimensional" on track and field. Finally, it allowed me to further my education while also running track as a professional.

And so I was set up for the best possible outcome. This was a new chapter on my life journey. It was also one I was excited to embark on. It's truly ironic how life tends to work. I started my athletic career playing football, expecting to play QB at LSU. From there, it was the NFL, stardom, money, everything of false value.

STARDUST DREAMS

Obviously, none of it panned out in that manner. In truth, it was best for it not to occur. While my dream of playing in the NFL will never happen, the dream of being a pro athlete is still alive. Albeit, in a much different sport with, sadly, less money involved. Undeniably, it was the best outcome I had hoped for to start this new chapter.

To make the adjustment to professional sports more manageable, I decided to refine my mechanics that summer. Having everything somewhat figured out allowed me time to focus on the more minor things. I was tired of hitting the hurdles because I was tired of hearing people comment on it. I also figured maybe changing things up could benefit me greatly. Much to my pleasure, my technique began refining in some areas.

The progress made was synonymous with the newfound mentality I had. It was my rookie season, but I wasn't a rookie in the game. At that point, I had been hurdling for 11 years. There was simply no excuse for some weaknesses my game had. I knew cleaning up my mechanics could be a great benefit.

That entire summer was essentially a transitional period. I knew it was time to leave LSU in the past. That also meant leaving certain people behind as well. Lupa pushing me away caused me to do the same to others, mainly LSU-related individuals. I was just ready to leave it all behind and start anew. I am not proud of pushing away certain LSU-affiliated people, especially friends who were still on the team. Yet, deep down, I knew I had to for whatever twisted reason.

It just felt like time to fight for my life. That included fighting for the dream of becoming a professional athlete. Also, fighting for what I wanted out of people in my life. I wanted to surround myself with people who made me better. I wanted to surround myself with individuals who truly wanted to see me succeed. But, most of all, I desired a romantic relationship with a girl not named "Lupa."

Towards the back end of summer, I managed the gull to ask a girl out on a date. She was someone I befriended during my time as an LSU athlete. In retrospect, going on a date with that girl was symbolic for many reasons. One reason was my willingness to leave Lupa, a very influential person, in the past. The second reason was to find an emotional bond with a girl not named "Lupa."

On that date, I remember a specific question the girl posed to me about my time as a college athlete. She asked, "Do you have any regrets"? It was quite the odd question, but it made me think of everything in a brief flash. From the first day, I walked through the halls at LSU, all the way to my final stride across the white line at Regionals. From the first day I greeted Lupa to the day we parted ways. From the first day of practice to the last plane ride home in LSU gear. I smiled and responded confidently, "nope, not a single one." Looking into her eyes, I realized that the next chapter of my life had already begun.

To summarize this entire chapter, my willingness to move forward defines everything. I needed growth to fearlessly retake control over my life. Admittedly, I still have a wide array of fears in my life. Truthfully, the fear regarding everything I've said is the fear of failure. My biggest fears include failing out of graduate school, wasting time running track, not being financially stable enough, being stuck in life, etc. There are many fears, none of which I have overcome just yet. Perhaps that is a good thing, as fear can often be the greatest motivator if we allow it. Fear can be very paralyzing, but it can also prompt us to move forward.

Being able to peer into the future is simply out of my ability as a human. With that being said, my faith is in the hands of the Lord. I am unsure how my future will unravel. However, I am confident I am on the right path. I don't know if I will gain prominence in track and field or if my road will lead to another career choice. No matter the outcome, I proved that I wasn't mentally or physically stuck.

    This is a new chapter in my life. Hopefully, it is the best one yet. I pray this chapter helps me grow as a man. No, as the King, I dream of becoming in the future. Right now, my feet are in the present. Wherever God may steer me, that is where I will walk, tall and proud, down this blessed starlit road. May fate be kind.

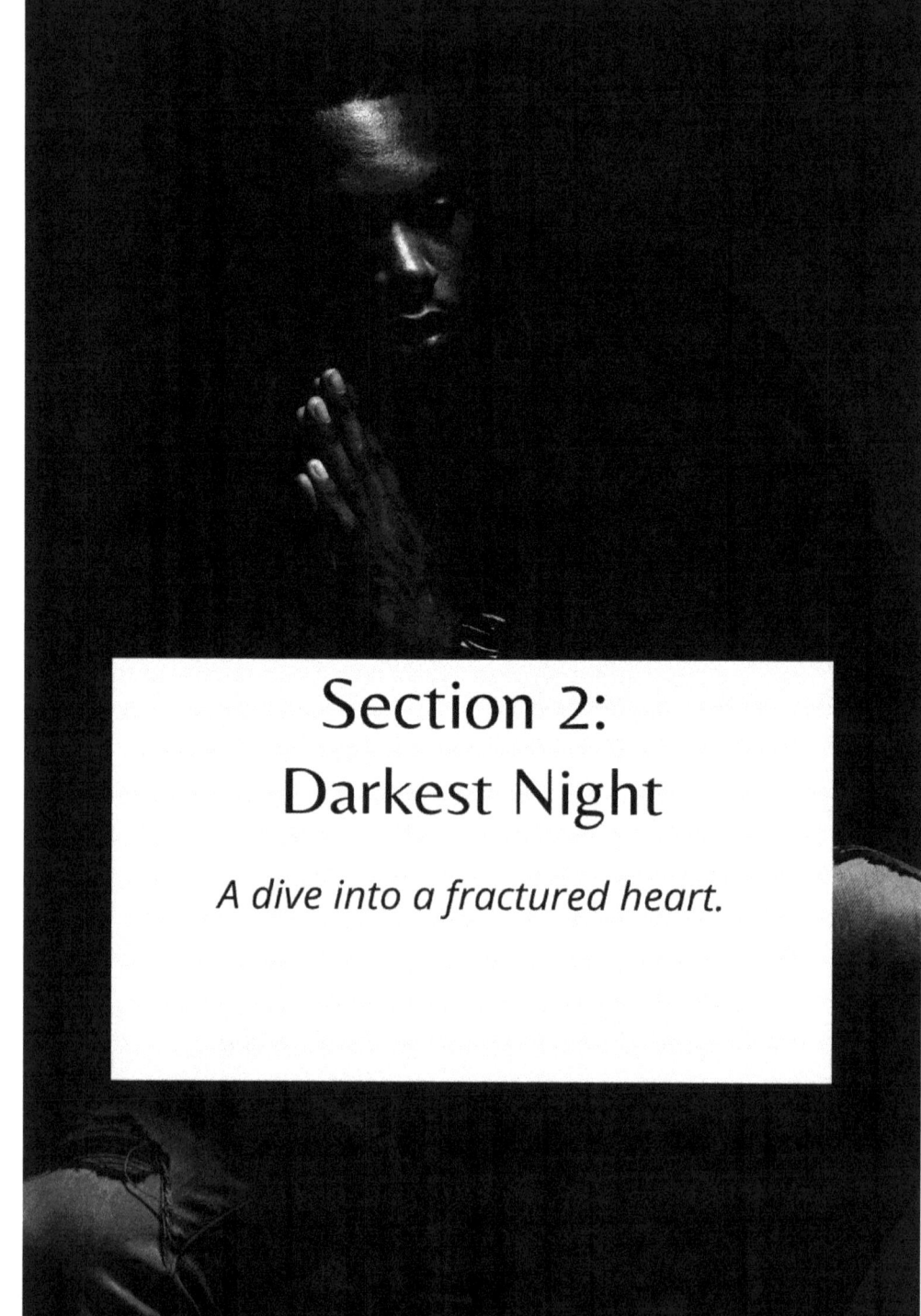

Section 2: Darkest Night

A dive into a fractured heart.

Chapter 4: Black Hole

CHAPTER IV: Black Hole

"Growing old and dying is what gives meaning and beauty to a human life. It is because we age and die that our lives have value and nobility."
  - *Koyoharu Gotouge,*
  [Kimestu no Yaiba 8]

It is fitting the name of this chapter is called "black hole." I have wanted to include a chapter such as this one for a long time. Every page of this chapter symbolically contains a piece of my soul. Not the piece most people may see, but rather the unseen and unknown. While I generally consider myself a good person, I have always struggled with my "darkness." Everyone has a dark side; such is human nature. My darkness, uniquely, can be defined as many things.

My darkness is something I haven't quite overcome yet but have learned to control with great success. The darkness in my heart is not something I want to eliminate, nor could I. Light will always cast shadows. To know good, one must know evil. With life comes death; with creation comes destruction. Duality has existed before the time of man and will continue to do so after.

To begin with, my entire life, I have often been a misunderstood individual. People often associate me with specific traits such as anger, obnoxiousness, overly optimistic, hard-working, intelligent, etc. All of which are very much true in some regard. However, behind all of that is something dark – apathy. In layman's terms, apathy means being unable to feel emotion. Feeling emotion is something I have always desired but never truly felt in any capacity besides rare moments of anger. The one feeling I have always sought above all others has been unconditional, non-transactional, legitimized love.

As a child, it was challenging to explore my emotions. Growing up in a military-centered family may result in emotions never being explored. Tears would be met with comments such as "grow up" or be dismissed entirely. Happy moments were not overly joyous occasions either. My hopes and dreams were constantly met with the limited expectations from my family to "join the military" instead. In so many ways, I adopted the military mindset. This also included the suppression of emotions.

The emotional talks were something I never had. It wasn't a question of love as I knew my family did love me. Yes, I have had disagreements with most members of my family. Yet, I knew deep down they did love me. But, it was almost as if emotions were something never explored. It was almost as if emotions were never meant to exist in forms besides anger to "keep the troops in check."

Even as an adult, I grew envious of people whose families appeared to support their goals unconditionally. At least from my point of view, that is what it seemed to be. For example, during my time in college, nobody in my family ever watched me compete in person. Over time, I stopped caring because it seemed as if my family didn't think much of me as an athlete. They didn't value me as a unique person besides a future military officer. At least, that is what I used to think. I never told my family how much it bothered me for them to limit me in such a fashion. Rather, I didn't know how to or if my disgruntlement even mattered to them.

Not knowing how to explore my emotions may have contributed to my apathy, even at a young age. My indifference has often caused me to view people as objects. It has also caused me to fear connections that would potentially develop. The need to keep friends and family at a distance became a necessity. Ignoring beautiful girls who would seemingly throw themselves at my feet became common.

People come and go, so there was little to no need for the temporary. People and emotions were seen as temporary by my twisted conscience. The scariest part is that I didn't care. I didn't care who I was hurting by keeping everyone at a distance. I wanted to be alone because I didn't want to build up something destined to crumble. I knew once it crumbled, so too would my heart.

The death of my mother in late 2018 broke me. In my head, I failed as a son. There was so much anger I held towards myself as a result. Persistence had always rewarded me, yet persistence didn't save my mother for some reason. Hours of researching and helping, yet none of it mattered.

My mother didn't lose her battle with dementia because she fought for years. However, I lost the battle with life because hers was handed to death. I couldn't save her, and it still haunts me to this very day. I was trying to fight for her and be the son she needed. I was even willing to fight death to extend her life longer. Yet, I still failed in saving and protecting her.

About a year after my mother's death, I experienced the death of my friendship with Lupa.

Although physical death wasn't involved this time, emotional death was. Lupa was the person I confided in once I received news of my mother's passing. I thought our bond could withstand anything, yet it vanished instantly. That was perhaps the turning point behind everything. It was when my apathy became stronger and more present.

For years after losing my mother and the friendship I held with Lupa, I struggled emotionally. Primarily with the overall value of human life. I know all things must perish, but the understanding I held was narrow-minded. If people and relationships were temporary, there had to be no value to life. I contemplated things such as love and family, deducing it was meaningless since they would cease to exist. Once they did expire, they were lost to time, almost as if it never existed. I thought to myself, "life is just an ephemeral hell."

Simply put, not being able to form meaningful connections often causes me to feel disconnected from life. I tried to learn through others what emotions were and perhaps understand what makes life so valuable. The disconnection has caused me to always be an outsider in some capacity, no matter the environment.

Due to being an outsider, I consider myself to have a different perspective from most. I view murder, rape, and other horrendous crimes as pointless violence. Even as a child, I often contemplated why people would harm others in such a vile way. I never understood why some people enjoy harming others for pleasure. Racism was another subject that condemned me to spend hours in meditation.

For another person to hate me because of my skin color was stupid. To add, people who shared my skin color demeaned me because of my speech. I never understood how people who "love" each other could say things to belittle each other. There were so many evils I saw and hated. It all felt pointless and made me view humans as vile creatures.

While I do love people, sometimes I find myself hating people. I'm not too fond of those who look down on the less fortunate. Maybe, I've always put myself in the shoes of those forsaken souls. Perhaps I've always viewed myself as a weakling. And so, the only way to not feel weak was to be unjustifiably angry. Back then, I held the twisted belief more anger equals more power, which equals more intimidation.

Anger is the prime contradiction to my apathy. Anger has always been the one emotion I've always felt. However, the anger I held over time led to hate. Whenever my anger would take over throughout my life, it would be coupled with hatred. As a result, both my anger and hatred towards many things grew.

For example, I have always felt anger from not reaching the ideal "athletic" pinnacle. The insecurity caused me to hate myself for any athletic shortcomings. However, it also motivated me to become stronger in an attempt to love myself. Another example would be the occurrence of my mother's passing. I felt anger toward the world and hatred toward myself for being powerless to change her fate.

Anger is a powerful emotion. It can be used for good and evil. It is no more dangerous than a raging storm but beneficial like a guiding breeze in the wind. My anger has caused me to do both unique and unbecoming things. But, what was the root of it all? Rather, who was I truly behind the anger and hatred? What were my anger and hatred truly aimed towards?

I sought psychological help in the latter part of 2020 during fall training for track. Initially, the weekly meetings with the therapist were geared toward coping with my broken friendship with Lupa. Yet, all those meetings started uncovering who I was, good and bad. It made me realize certain things about myself and the gifts inside which were ignored. Most importantly, it made me more loving of myself.

Going to therapy made me realize the root of my anger –myself. I held so much anger towards myself yet blamed "life." I blamed life for the family I was given and the limited athletic potential it seemed I appeared to have. I blamed life for taking away my mother, Lupa, and other people I had grown to care about, be it to death or split paths. But, most of all, I blamed life for making me weak as I could do nothing to change anything. All of which was reflective of a past version of me.

It was the first time in my life emotions were explored. Actually, it was the first time I realized other emotions besides anger resided in me. The slow realizations I had with my rage made me want to change. No, it made me realize I had the power to change. However, the change had to start with the person responsible for everything, myself. Putting this responsibility on myself wasn't necessarily playing a "blame game." It meant, for the first time in my life, I had to accept myself for all my shortcomings and achievements.

By accepting myself, I realized for the majority of my life, I never felt human. The enjoyments most had as children, I never got to experience. I often viewed myself as an outsider from others as well. I never truly learned the expression of emotions until my mid-20s. Finally, it felt as if everything I bottled up was starting to come out.

The "bottle of emotions" was agitated for years yet poured out so peacefully. It made me realize how blessed I was to be alive. It also made me realize that although my past wasn't ideal, it doesn't mean my future won't be glorious. However, I had to remain in the present, not look too far forward or too far behind. "Yesterday is history, tomorrow is a mystery, today is a gift, that is why it is called the present," as an old Chinese proverb states.

STARDUST DREAMS

Going to therapy made me feel human. It also made me begin to value human life. Instead of being dismissive of people, I started becoming more open. Albeit, while still protecting my heart, since it is the source of my soul's flow. I stopped seeing people as objects and more so as unique creatures. Our lives are fragile, yet that does not mean it lacks value. It only takes one ember to set a forest ablaze. Even the smallest forms of life have a purpose in this experience we call "existence."

This was driven home with the passing of an old childhood love interest. I will refer to this resting soul as W, my old friend. W and I met one fateful 4th of July night in 2014. I had just graduated high school and was stressed with college on the horizon. W was experiencing the same stresses of the life transitions. She was just like me in the ways that mattered, age included. However, she was different in those same ways as well. I became immediately fond and attracted to W, almost faster than a speeding bullet.

As time progressed, the infatuation became a respectable friendship, which did fade over time. However, it wasn't until 2022 I heard news regarding W. To my shock, the news was of her unfortunate passing. I was paralyzed with disbelief, yet didn't know why. W and I stopped speaking to each other in 2016. But, we both still wanted to see the other person succeed. Upon hearing the news, tears poured from my eyes, unintentionally. I didn't know why I was crying, nor could I control it. It was almost as though my soul was weeping instead of me intentionally creating tears.

While W dealt with her demons, in my opinion, she won. She gave birth to two children, graduated college, and was even engaged. She was overcoming the struggles life had placed on her. Her life mattered because of her impact on others, including me. Her passing hit home because there were so many things I wanted to say to W in our old age. I wanted to tell her how proud I was of the woman she had become. I appreciated her life because it had so much value. May her soul rest in the peace she found, the peace she deserved.

Perhaps the perfect way to summarize this chapter is for it to be an "exploration" into the abyss of my soul. While my dream is to become a King in my own right, learning about emotion is essential. Even as I write this book, I am still discovering what it means to be human. That's because, in my opinion, being human is having emotion. Not just that, being able to explore and express those emotions. Emotions such as love, anger, sadness, and joy give beauty to the fleeting human life.

There is no need to feel emotionless anymore. Life does have value; it always has, it always will. I won't act as if I don't still struggle with my emotions. Certain things still haunt my soul. But, learning what it means to be human, to have emotion, etc., is part of my journey to become a King. After all, a king is guided by his heart. What lies in his heart is a reflection of his soul.

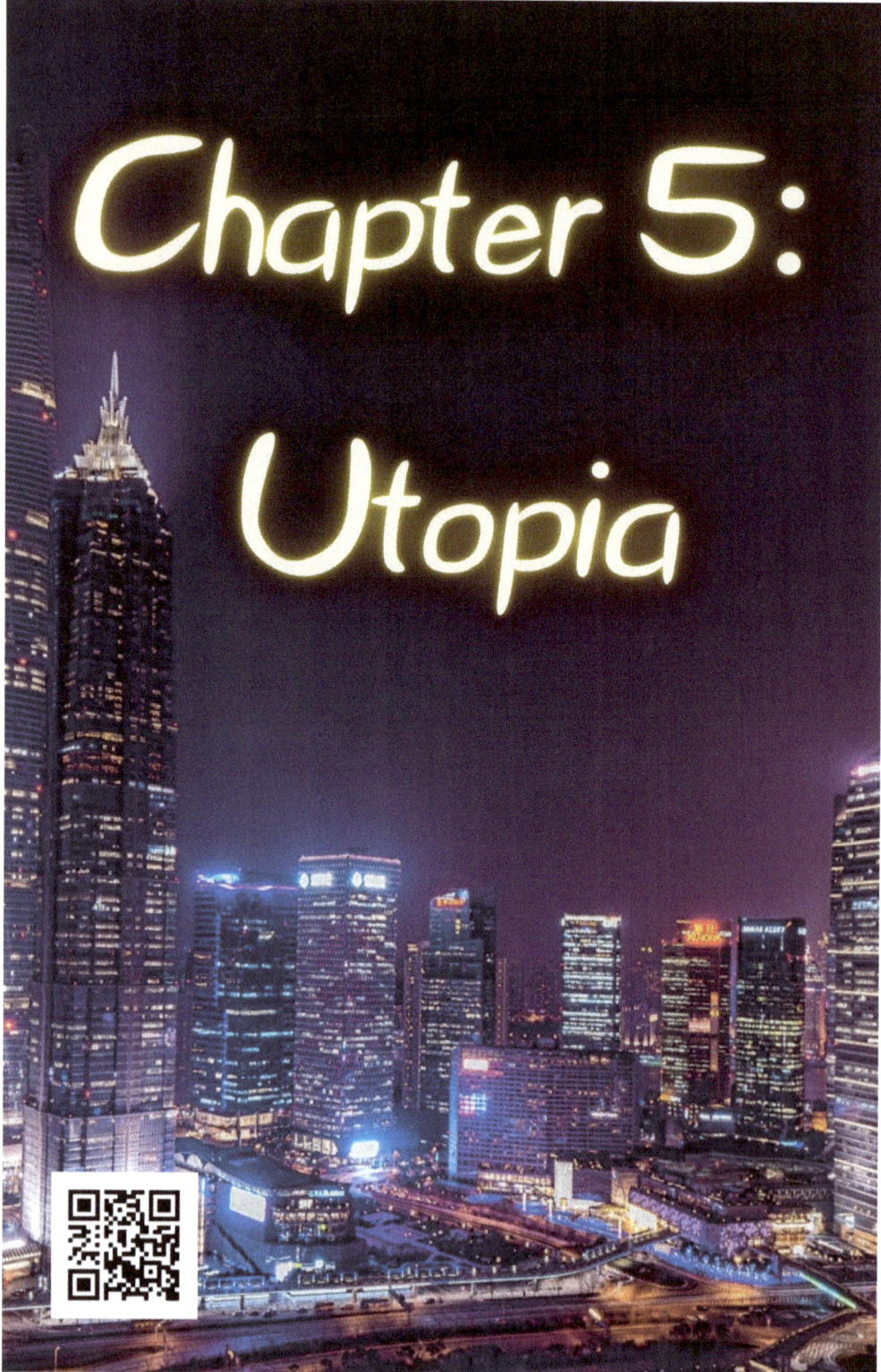

CHAPTER V: Utopia

"In this life, you will be met with both admiration and abuse from others. How others choose to view you is a choice only they can make. You cannot make it for them. All that matters is that you hold firm to your own values."
― *Unknown*

In a utopia, everything is supposed to be perfect. It is supposed to be the ideal society. Rather, it is a world of fantasy one can only dream of. It is a world of fantasy based on reality. In my utopia, everyone loves me. It is a world I created out of my long-sought desire to feel loved.

To have people cheer my name in constant celebration and admiration. "The glorious King Arthur," I imagined they would say. Unfortunately, this world is one of fiction as it can never truly exist. I often awaken from this world of fantasy with the disappointments of reality.

"Sorry, we only cover accomplished athletes." Yes, those were the words once uttered to me. About two weeks later, those words were followed with "your book isn't good enough for our news site." I almost forgot to mention the 2-star review one person gave my first book on Amazon. The review was damning because only one person felt the need to review it with such criticism. There were many criticisms and multiple instances of rejection that followed suit. It made me feel as though my first book was terrible. Rather, my story wasn't remarkable enough in the eyes of others.

    Why was I beginning to think this? After all, many of these instances of rejection and criticism were from smaller groups of people. Even close friends didn't seem to like the first book, which was reflected in their overall support. There were instances when I had to ask my friends to re-post my book on social media. I never understood why my friends didn't seem to reciprocate the support. More prominent news publications such as Spikes Magazine, the Baton Rouge Advocate, and The Daily Reveille (LSU's official school newspaper) felt my story was amazing. Because of my book, I even formed relationships with the reporters who worked at those respective news organizations. Yet, why was I still so concerned with the minority and their opinions?

Due to the conflict regarding my first book, I almost gave up writing in general. Thankfully, I didn't give into the negative thoughts. Before starting this second book, I had to place myself in the right mindset. There was only one way to approach such. That way included addressing my insecurities. Everyone in the world is insecure about at least one thing. Although those insecurities might not arise to the surface, they are hidden within. While I am a very proud, strong individual, I have the insecurity of inferiority.

Growing up, I always felt as if I was viewed as "inferior." Attending all-white private schools for most of my life was not good for my psyche, being an African-American. I remember feeling below others in my earlier years due to my skin color. It was impossible to avoid the negativity I was subjugated to. The boys would tease me because of my skin color. The girls never looked my way due to me not "fitting their standards." There were days I would return from elementary school to stare in a mirror. "My nose and lips are too big, that's what everyone says," I thought.

These thoughts were always soothed with my mother's loving words. "I'm beautiful, you're my son, that makes you handsome." Looking back on that, my mother was right in every single way. Simply put, I am sexy and I know it. Ironically, now I consider myself to be quite the narcissist. Sometimes, I stare in the mirror in amazement and appreciate my amazing looks. I credit both my parents for that. As such, thank you, Arthur Price Jr and Joycelyn Price.

Aside from facial features, my dismay was geared towards other physical attributes, mainly around the stomach area. "I don't have abs like everyone else, does that mean I'm fat?" Even as an adult, these words still find their way into my head. People have always criticized my physique, especially in the track world. Growing up, I was never a "skinny twig," as some people referred to themselves as. Yet, I was never genuinely overweight, though others considered me as such.

I was always a strong, bulking, healthy person. Yet, for high school football, I was deemed to be underweight. It prompted me to "bulk up" while consuming everything in sight. "I have to get bigger" was the singular thought in my mind. It was a thought that didn't originate as my own. Instead, it was a thought that became my own because of the opinions of others. Once I gave up football, the weight carried over into track.

"You're fat as shit," one teammate said during my first year on the LSU track team. That same year, there was even a rainy day where we all took pictures in the weight room, shirtless. Because of the "fat" comment, I kept my shirt on in shame.

That entire first season as an LSU athlete was an eye-opener. Everyone was progressing, while I wasn't. I was running 10.9 in the 100m dash, a feat many elite female sprinters can achieve. I decided to change everything and focus wholeheartedly on losing weight. The insecurity I felt about my physique prompted a tremendous change.

After losing 20lbs, I became an elite athlete in my own right. The change was beneficial, but it was done out of insecurity. The weight loss was also a result of the motivation to be a better athlete. Everything worked out the way it was meant to occur in this scenario. Yet, even as a professional athlete, my physique is still criticized.

During the first training cycle as a pro, there was an instance I was referred to as "fat" once more. How could that be so? While I was a bit heavier than usual, all my weightlifting maxes went up significantly. So, was I really "fat" or just a tad out of shape from not running during the summer? Was my body weight increase due to pure fat or the muscle I gained? Did others view me as "fat" because I love wearing comfortable, baggy clothes?

Questions such as those posed prior tend to make me paranoid due to my insecurities, body-wise. It even caused me to overanalyze my last season as a collegiate athlete. I was beginning to think the subpar final season was due to excess body weight. I was a tad skinner in 2019 when I became an All-American. However, I felt as if my body had gained more power. In 2020, I PR'd in the 60m hurdles weighing about 3lbs heavier while having a damaged hamstring.

"Maybe I should change my hurdling so I don't hit them as often," I concluded. After all, I've been criticized heavily due to constantly hitting hurdles during a race. The criticisms regarding my hurdle technique weren't heard in the breakout 2019 season. When I fell at Nationals that same year, the rumblings of "if you didn't hit hurdles…" began. Falling at nationals caused me to spend years re-evaluating my hurdle technique. I didn't want to fall again, nor did I want to hear people's critics. I found myself adapting the techniques others would use to succeed, disregarding my own. I was essentially rejecting the uniqueness God had given me by doing so.

There is a reason why I do tend to hit hurdles. My take-off is much closer than it should be relative to my height. In layman's terms, I hurdle as if I am 6"3 instead of hurdling like the 6"0 athlete I am. According to some people, due to this "technical inferiority," I should have never been able to be successful as a hurdler. Yet, I've gone on to run blistering times.

In addition, I've only ever fallen twice during my entire career. Of course, falling is something every hurdler will experience at some point. But, according to some, I should've fallen more because I took off "too close." Perhaps my take-off is right where it needs to be. Heck, hurdlers with "perfect" technique have fallen many more times than I have.

Unfortunately, others surpassed me during my two-year struggles after falling at nationals. It did not sit well with me. In my mind, there were zero reasons why others were surpassing me. I often found myself depressed and contemplating whether or not track was worth it. My last year on the team was filled with comments about being "too old."

It was almost as if those opinions of being "old" became the viewpoint I thought of myself. Funnily enough, those thoughts started manifesting physically through various aches and pains throughout my final collegiate season. Those factors caused me to think I was just a "washed up" athlete in his mid-20s. In actuality, the mid-20s are usually an athlete's prime. Yet, I allowed the environment around me to intoxicate my mind.

Still today, there are various unimportant things which intoxicate my mind. Social media used to be a significant part of my life, athletically speaking. I used to put so much worth into social media. I thought the number of followers or attention on social media was indicative of a person's value. For example, during the summer of 2021, I tried my damn hardest to get verified on Instagram. Yet, as I write this memoir, I am still not verified on the platform. I felt so much animosity during that summer due to not having that "prestigious blue check" next to my name on social media. The "badge of authenticity" which symbolizes I am a "relevant" person in the eyes of Instagram.

It wasn't until after countless attempts to get verified, I realized something vital. It was stupid to care about a simple "blue check." It would have never defined me as an athlete, in all honesty. I've been in the media multiple times, have run at various big-time meets, and even wrote an entire book. So, in reality, just because Instagram didn't think I was relevant does not mean I am not an amazing, important person.

So, how does everything I said up to this point come full circle, you may ask. To put it simply, if you try to please everyone, you will always disappoint yourself in the process. It is impossible to please other humans due to our innate nature. Humans will never be satisfied with others, nor with themselves. The latter of which is why we compare ourselves to others. People will always place limitations on others. This occurs for various reasons such as jealousy, doubt, etc. In this world, everyone's a critic, not just of themselves but of others as well.

It is so damn hard to deal with other people and their negativity. The main reason is because humans naturally desire love. As people, we want to feel love from others. The love we feel from the people around us makes us feel important. However, this should never be the case as it is very unhealthy. While the people around us need to give love, it should not impact how we view ourselves.

The moments of insecurity throughout this chapter are examples of times I didn't love myself. From the insecurities about my facial features to the pettiness of wanting a blue check on Instagram. All those moments of insecurity resulted from allowing the opinions of others to dictate my thoughts. I did not have the inner confidence I possess now during those situations.

Some news organizations scoffed at my first book. So then, was I a terrible writer? According to other kids, I was ugly. So then, by default, was I? A select few have called me "fat" because I didn't fit their subjective norm of body types. Therefore, was my weight truly an issue? Others often criticize my athletic abilities. So then, was I athletically inadequate? Instagram didn't think I was "relevant" enough to have a blue check next to my name. Therefore, am I not important in the world?

The confident, resounding answer to those questions is "NO." Why? Well, because those are the opinions others possess. While I have my obvious flaws, only I know all of them. If other people truly knew me, they would speak on all my flaws, not just those they see or think may exist. In the end, it is their own opinion. People are fully entitled to have their opinions. It does not mean I have to agree with their very shite opinions and perceptions.

On that same note, it is appropriate to give my thanks. I am thankful for the people who doubted me. I am thankful for every person that rejected me because I wasn't "good enough" in their eyes. I am also thankful that I didn't allow those same people to destroy my future. I am thankful for rising back up every time I allowed others to tear me down. I am thankful for those who hate me because it led to loving myself even more. To those same people, as famous actress Polly Holiday once said, "y'all can kiss my grits."

Listen clearly, for this is my declaration. I am a handsome, young, educated African-American man. I am a fantastic author and will continue to publish literary works. I am healthy in all ways, physical, mental, spiritual, and emotional. I am a great athlete on the path to becoming legendary. I am talented in many disciplines and will continue to grow as a human. So, don't ever doubt me in any fashion. I am perfectly imperfect in every way that matters.

Just because people may not view me in the way I desire does not mean I am less than a person. In this world, things such as fame are man-given. Fame comes and goes just like a windy breeze. How people view me is no longer how I view myself. I unconditionally love myself with one hundred percent guaranteed confidence in myself. After all, a king has to be confident.

If people can't see how amazing I am, it's their opinion. It is not "their loss" because I am not an object to be had by others. I am a king worthy of the appreciation I give myself daily. As long as I have myself and my dreams, I have true wealth. Now, how's that for a chapter?

Even as I write this book, I am still discovering what it means to be human. That's because, in my opinion, being human is having emotion. Not just that, being able to explore and express those emotions. Emotions such as love, anger, sadness, and joy give beauty to the fleeting human life.

There is no need to feel emotionless anymore. Life does have value; it always has, it always will. I won't act as if I don't still struggle with my emotions. Certain things still haunt my soul. But, learning what it means to be human, to have emotion, etc., is part of my journey to become a King. After all, a king is guided by his heart. What lies in his heart is a reflection of his soul.

CHAPTER 6:

NIGHTMARES IN DREAMLAND

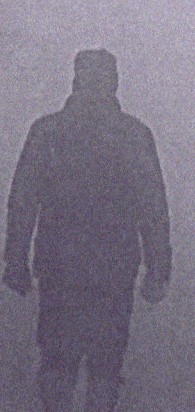

CHAPTER VI: Nightmares in Dreamland

"Every dream as a process and a price tag. Those wo embrace the process and pay the price, live the dream. Those who don't, just dream."
- Jeremy Riddle

It is hard to be a dreamer. Being a dreamer means others will outcast you. It means you will be doubted by the same people who were afraid to live their dreams. It is okay to be frightened, but your fears cannot paralyze you. Nor can you be paralyzed with the fears others will try to place into your head.

The expectations for yourself must be higher than the limitations others place on you. If you are confident in yourself, that is all that matters. Confidence is of the utmost importance, so please protect it. There will be moments of failure and success. But, through it all, the pain you feel will be worth it one day.

As a dreamer myself, I've had to endure much physical toll. In the years of being an athlete, I've suffered many injuries. Some injuries still ache from time to time. One of the most visible injuries is on my left pinkie finger. In my senior year of high school, I fractured it during competition from football. At the time, the injury was damning because of my position.

I was a running back who played a tad bit of receiver in the slot position. In short, I needed my hands to function properly. It was senior year, and I struggled to get on the field due to the NFL talent ahead of me. I remember taking painkillers every day, wrapping half of my left hand in bandages. I did anything and everything to make the most out of whatever chance I had on the field.

One of the main reasons I left football was my realization regarding injuries. As long as there's someone behind you, fans, coaches, etc., don't care if you're injured. To that same notion, most only care if you're healthy, playing on the field, scoring touchdowns for their team. Was risking life-alternating injuries worth a materialistic piece of hardware or millions of dollars? In the most unselfish of events, it's for loved ones. Yet, when I look down at my left pinkie, I often ask myself one question. "What am I struggling for, and how much more do I need to struggle?"

My past playing football "toughened" me up to where bumps and bruises don't bother me. As a hurdler, one has to be tough, especially considering the nature of the event:

1. Running over a barrier (no matter the height) usually leads to cuts and bruises anyway.
2. There's always a chance you will fall. In fact, it is a guarantee that every hurdler has fallen at least once.
3. A hurdler must be aggressive, even with the risks in mind.

This brings me to my mental apparatus. After falling at NCAA Nationals in 2019, I became timid. I am slowly returning to the aggressive mindset I once had. Physically, I am strong, yet mentally I need to improve. My mind is often the most significant obstacle to overcome, especially with hurdling. Physically, I've done it thousands of times. My body remembers how to hurdle as if it was instinctual. Yet, when one misfire occurs, my mind goes into "repair" mode rather than dismiss it as a minor error.

A prime example of this is in my hurdle technique. To start things off, I am a very aggressive hurdler. I don't mind hitting hurdles. Although, it is not my goal to do so during a race. There are often times I don't even feel myself hitting the hurdles at all. In reality, I could be limiting myself by hitting the hurdles. In contrast, perhaps hitting hurdles doesn't have much of a factor, for me at least. I've run my fastest races hitting every hurdle, just as I've run my slowest races, trying to avoid them.

STARDUST DREAMS

I am not advocating for my style to be implemented. What I am saying is my hurdle style is unique to me. It is a style I used to become an All-American and ranked top 8 at one point in the USA for my event. It is a style which gave me the chance to be a competitor in the 2021 Olympic Trials in Eugene, Oregon. Every hurdler has their style, just like I do.

Since every hurdler has their style, why did I ever feel the need to change mine? The answer is simple – to make other people happy. Truthfully, with the time I spent trying to "fix" my technique, I could have been embracing the God-given one I had. I could have built upon strengths, like my lightning-fast start. Instead of being self-damaging by doing what others thought I should've done. Mentally, I let people in that should've never had a place in my head.

The harsh critics about my hurdling style almost caused me to quit the event in its entirety. Back then, I should've listened more to my heart than to the voices of others. It isn't easy to do so, especially when those voices are from loved ones. Often, we listen to our loved ones more than other people because we want to believe our family, friends, etc., have our best interests in mind. It is important to remember, people will constantly critique you based on their perceptions.

For example, some of my closest people don't think much of me as a track athlete. I feel it in their support or lack thereof. Likewise, I never felt some of my friends or family members celebrated my athletic accomplishments. I've had people scoff at my passion for track and field in some cases. Lupa was a prime example of such doubts and negativity. "I can't believe you think it's your destiny to win a championship."

Hearing those words from her lips was a bit painful. Lupa misinterpreted my mindset because she viewed me being a one-dimensional person, goal-wise. There has been time involving family regarding negativity as well. I've had family members suggest quitting sports in general on numerous occasions. I even found myself wanting to quit running to appease them.

With the opinions of friends and family, along with the words Lupa once uttered to me, I lost my passion for running for three years. Yes, I was allowing the outside noises to take over. But, those outside noises were from people I trusted. I figured they would only want the best for me. I just thought they would see things I was too oblivious to notice. But, those same voices were the same ones that slowly made me rethink my dreams. I was beginning to let people kill my dreams.

Financial hardships have also caused me to rethink my dreams. During my entire time as an undergraduate student, my financial situation was always murky. Before becoming a member of the LSU track and field team, I was a regular college student. My father's veteran benefits were a blessing to help start my college education. I also received additional aid such as the Pell grant, pelican promise, etc.

However, all of those "blessings" were timed and privileged. I didn't have the motivation to find a job because all of my tuition was already paid. The refund checks I received were also enough to manage for six months since I didn't have to pay bills at a time. Admittedly, having the money available caused me to have no ambition to make money. Even though I was doing well in school, I could have done more outside of school besides athletics. My younger self was still very much green in all matters of finance.

Once the veteran benefits and grants dried up, I had to turn to other sources of aid, loans. Most college athletes have zero loan debt. Unfortunately, I do not fall into this category. Although I was on the roster, I was only a walk-on. It is very rare for college walk-ons to receive assistance from a program. Most college walk-ons have to work jobs outside of school and athletics to make a living.

Fortunately, in my second year, I was blessed enough to receive a track scholarship from LSU.

However, even the scholarships eventually waned as my time being a collegiate athlete ended. In anticipation of this, I began to work teacher assistant jobs to help pay for finances during my last year of collegiate athletics. I still work as a teacher assistant for Arizona State University. It is a remote position, but it doesn't pay as much as my assistantship job at LSU. Having maturity helped me realize I could/need to work more jobs. But, this has caused overlapping conflicts in me.

The first is finding a job that doesn't feel like a job. I very much enjoy being a teacher's assistant. To be realistic, it isn't a job I can genuinely rely on since it is only part-time. Grading papers and helping students learn unique skills is very rewarding. Sadly, it doesn't keep my lights on. I am very qualified for multiple positions relating to STEM. I graduated from LSU with a major in psychology and a minor in chemistry.

STARDUST DREAMS

My goal after professional sports is to do research of some form relating to neurology. Such was a motivator to apply at various psychology clinics. Yet, during the application and interview processes, a moment of clarity occurred. "I don't want these jobs," I thought. Working part-time in a clinic would be fun and needed to further my career. For some reason, it was as if God told me to wait for better.

My patience often conflicts with the need to feel progression. At the time of writing this, I am 26 years old. I'm very young, very healthy, and haven't even started balding yet. Still, I often feel the need to rush everything. The need to feel "settled" with a promising career, be it as a professional track athlete or as a scientist. Now more than ever, I'm investing time into my professional track career.

I am essentially running until I run out of time, pun intended. Being 26 years old, I am in my prime. My prime is not something I will have as a 35-year-old. Science can wait in the future; the present is reserved for sports. Although, I often ask myself how much I am willing to limit myself.

Could the time for track be re-channeled towards something more rewarding? Although a shoe company does not sponsor me, I have partnered with Adidas as a brand associate. The deal enables me to receive items with the condition of posting them on social media. That arrangement doesn't pay as handsome as most. Nonetheless, it is still something of value.

"Is any of this even worth it?", has echoed many times in my mind. Such voices are usually followed by "What is my dream?" Even having thoughts like, "Is there something else I should be doing? All these questions and more were reflective of the self-doubt I subjugated myself to. The self-hell I put myself in caused me to undergo a journey of reflection. As a child, my dream was to play in the NFL. As a collegian, my dream was to win an individual championship.

STARDUST DREAMS

Both of which never occurred, nor will they ever. Both of those facts I've accepted and have since moved on. But, as a professional athlete, what is the next step? Most readers would assume the next step to be winning a professional title, becoming an olympian, etc. While readers would guess correctly, those are only short-term goals. So, after those short-term goals, what comes next?

My ultimate dream is to become a "king" in my own right. But, the questions of "how" are often followed by my self-imposed doubts. Those same self-doubts are things I struggle with daily. Self-doubts are a result of letting outside forces affect our internal selves. Your soul is your sanctuary, the place you must protect at all costs. When you feel yourself falling deeper into the pit of fear and anxiety, catch yourself and rise above.

Once again, it is hard to be a dreamer. Being a dreamer is exceptionally hard because I haven't truly defined my dream other than "being a king ." In reference to my last book, I view my life journey as a version of kingly majesty. Having something nobody can achieve, nor will do so after my time has passed. The pressure from others is something which shouldn't be underestimated.

Toning out the outside noises can be very difficult. The pressure of feeling behind in life can be suffocating as well. You will spend countless hours stressed while comparing yourself to peers. Most of all, the pressures we often place on ourselves are the hardest to overcome. We are never satisfied with the blessed moments, always anxiously looking toward the future.

Amid all the pressures surrounding us, always remember one thing. Your destiny does not lie in the hands of others. Your future will always lie within your own hands. You have the power to change the winds of fate. In that regard, don't be afraid to raise your flag and set sail. If we had everything figured out, life would be very dull. If we won every single time, we wouldn't know the pain of loss. The feeling of losing wouldn't prompt us to become better individuals.

On that path of self-growth, we often learn more about ourselves. So, always strive for greatness and never give up. I'm not saying it will be easy because it won't. You must be willing to cry and bleed. You must also be ready to be doubted, including by loved ones. You can't be afraid of going against the grain. It is your life, destiny, and dream; do not be deterred. If it matters to you, it has priceless value. So, to all my dreamers, I impart one final piece of motivation. Keep your eyes on the sky and your heart in the stars.

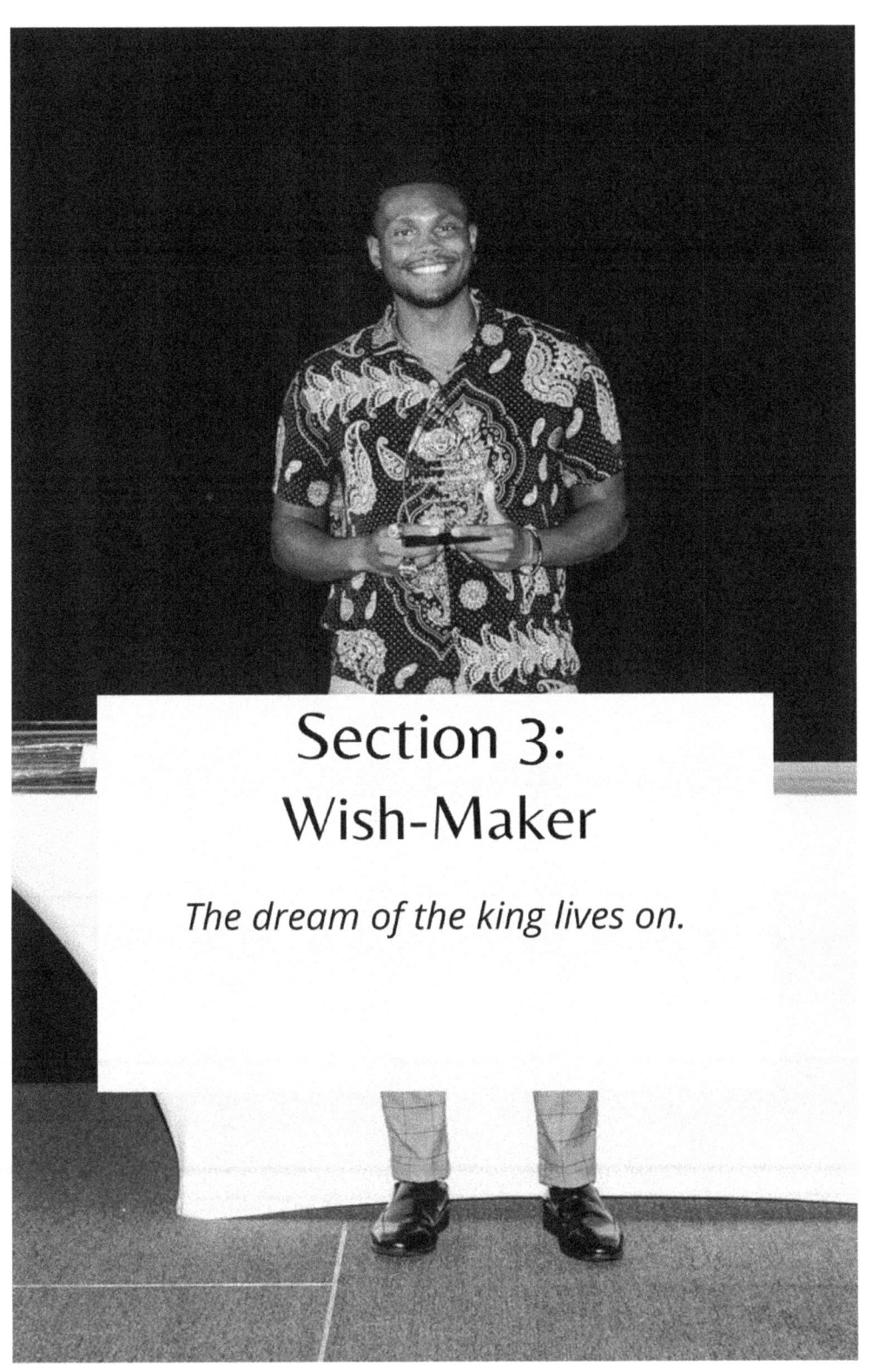

Section 3: Wish-Maker

The dream of the king lives on.

Chapter 7:

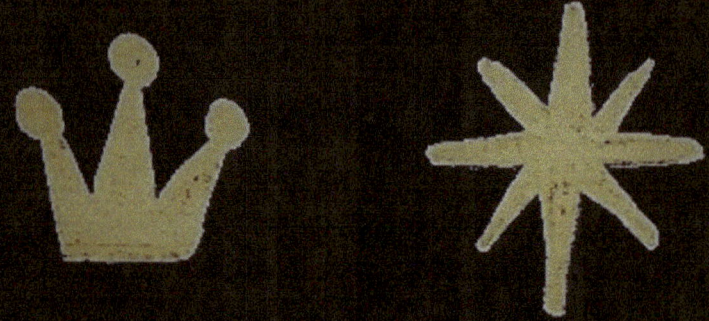

STARGAZER

CHAPTER VII: Stargazer

"Keep your eyes on the sky and your heart in the stars."
- Arthur C. Price III

The hardest part of writing is not knowing what to write about. Everyone's story is unique in its own way. However, not everyone can tell their story. The ability to write a masterpiece is a skill not all possess. Perhaps, I am one of those individuals. Yet, I am still compelled to write these words on a page and tell my story.

After all, life is about taking the first step. As humans, we must have confidence and faith to take the first step toward our dreams. The ground where our foot will land is unknown. We are stepping into an ominous, dark abyss, away from the comfortable light we bathed in. We do not know what lies ahead, but we must have confidence and faith; it will be better than the place we are leaving.

Such is the case from the day I felt my truly life began. It is a phenomenon I cannot explain but can detail vividly. Perhaps that was the day my brain began to function correctly. I remember waking up one cold October day at the tender age of five. I was in my bed, wearing Winnie the Pooh pajamas. It was as if I didn't experience the past day firsthand but knew I lived through it. It felt as if I was waking up from a dream or perhaps started living in one.

I took the first step out of my bed and was immediately bathed in the sun's light radiating from the window. The light's warmth protected me from what was an otherwise cold environment. I smelled food cooking in the kitchen and hurried towards the scent. As early as I could remember, breakfast had always been my favorite meal. The aroma of bacon grease, fried eggs, and fresh pancakes on a griddle was one I always associated happiness with.

My father was in the kitchen cooking my breakfast. My father also prepared hot chocolate with all the fixings to my excitement. My father was always the main chef in the house. As with all chefs, they take their kitchens as seriously as their foods. One of my father's rules was no eating allowed after 9 PM. The "closed kitchen" rule did make sense as my father wanted to start cooking in a clean kitchen every morning. Strict rules like these were standard from my father because he was in the military.

After sitting down to a complete breakfast feast in front of me, I was greeted by my mother, who told me a new episode of Big Brother was coming on later that day. My mother was a young, beautiful, talented woman. She was also a well-renowned teacher throughout the private school system. It just so happened that she was also a teacher for the upper grades at my school, St. Louis King of France. However, while some may see that as an advantage, it was the opposite for me. If I were to get in trouble at school, she would be the first to know. To add, seeing my mother around the school and having her blow me kisses was something I didn't value at the time.

Being a young boy, all I cared about was dirt, bugs, and toys, as did my fellow male classmates. Things such as love and girls were considered gross. I didn't want to catch "cooties," and lovey-dovey stuff wasn't manly. It was a toxic mentality fitting for my age and one I shared with most boys at the time. However, at home, I felt loved not just by her but also by my father. It was this day, one I remember so vividly and dreamy, that I felt loved.

Before leaving for school, I sat down with my father to watch a military movie. Back then, my father and I commonly watched movies like those. I didn't know what was going on in most of those movies. But that didn't matter as I spent time with my father while watching epic battle scenes.

Ironically, that same day, we watched one of my favorite movies to date.

The movie was called "*The Man in the Iron Mask.*" It featured Leonardo DiCaprio as the main star. DiCaprio played the fictional twin brother of King Louis of France. In the movie, the royal family hid the twin brother of Louis to prevent a future family clash for the throne. As a result, the unfortunate brother was locked up and forced to wear an iron mask to conceal his identity. The one scene I remembered from that movie is still, to this day, a favorite of mine.

The twin brother who donned the iron mask led the musketeers who helped free him into battle. The men charged toward the king of France and his gunmen while epic music played. The king ordered his men to shoot, much to their dismay. Having respect for the legendary musketeers, the king's gunmen fired without looking at their targets. Once the smoke clouds cleared, the king's twin brother in the iron mask nor the musketeers were injured.

STARDUST DREAMS

Seeing the "charge" scene before school gave me chills. I thought to myself, "it would be amazing to be the king that led the legendary musketeers into battle." Although it was just a movie, the majesty the man in the iron mask and the musketeers displayed was something to marvel at. Finally, the film ends with the twin brother taking over the throne with the help of the musketeers, taking upon the title of "King of France." Admittedly, the movie would make any five-year-old want to become a King.

At the conclusion of the movie, it was time to leave for school. The alarm to leave for school was always my mother's yell to "get in the damn car." On the way to school, I kept replaying the "charge" scene, imagining myself as the man in the iron mask. I was daydreaming about a world I felt comfortable in. But, alas, the daydream ended the moment I arrived at school.

At school, I was the only one of my kind. Being the only black kid in my class was something

I didn't consider due to childhood innocence. I was much different than the other kids in more ways than naught. Even at the earliest of ages, I was unique in that I stood out in the crowd. Perhaps I was a rose among weeds or the lone weed in a garden of roses. Either way, as early as I could remember, I felt alone amongst crowds while being the most notable one.

After my mother signed me into school for the day, I remember being greeted by the girl I had a crush on at the time. A beautiful blonde-haired, blue-eyed, hyper-active girl who was missing her two front teeth, I found myself swooning over at the time. Ironically enough, that same blonde-haired girl was my first official crush. I didn't know the feeling at the time, being so young, nor did I understand it. The butterflies in my stomach, sweaty hands, and awkward one-word answers were the typical first crush things.

She grabbed my hand, pulling me to the classroom where everyone was playing with the toys they snuck in from their homes. My hands were sweating with anxiety, and my smile was from ear to ear. I was eager to be a part of the group and play with toys I had never seen before. I was never the one to be considered as a "ring-leader" of the group growing up. I was always too timid and awkward to ever stand out.

My one redeeming quality was being considered the "cutest" boy by all of my female teachers. The girls in my classroom strangely thought the same. So cute, one of my teachers would grandmotherly kiss me on my forehead every day when my mother dropped me off. My mother didn't have a problem with it. Actually, she took credit for "gifting the world with a cutie." I was the "baby" of the classroom, as most of the female gender described me back then.

Once my blonde-haired crush brought me to the classroom, one of the boys called me over to show off his LEGO collection. Quickly pulling away from my crush, I ran towards the call of my name.

The first thing my socially awkward self noticed was the LEGO figure of a king wearing a crown. I asked the boy if I could play with it, to which he handed it to me without reply. I was ecstatic, as I had never had a toy quite like it.

I remember playing with the figurine the entire day. I didn't pay attention to anything or anybody. I even ignored my crush, who wanted me to color with her. As the LEGO figure, I imagined re-enacting the "charge" scene from "*Man in the Iron Mask.*" I was the king, leading my warriors into battle against an overwhelming army. The odds weren't in our favor, yet my men still trusted me to lead them to victory. Sadly, the world of imagination I created crumbled once it was time to give the boy back his toy.

On the ride home after school, I asked my mother if she could buy me a toy like the LEGO figurine I played with. "Ask Santa baby, 'cause I don't have the money," was her comical, albeit expected response. I then looked out my window towards the twilight sky and noticed a star. "Momma, do dreams really come true if you wish on a star?" My mother, fatigued from an entire day of teaching, replied with a simple "yes." I thought to myself, maybe if I wished upon that same star, I could get the LEGO toy before Christmas. Perhaps wishing upon that same star would make me become a real-life King.

Later that night, I watched the new episode of big brother with my mother. Fading back into my fantasy land, I began contemplating what kind of king I would be. "Would I be the king everyone kisses up to, or would I be the King everyone hates?" Being so young, I thought about the glorious result, yet never the most important things. Things such as "how will I become a king, or what does it mean to become a King?"

In reality, all I wanted was to stand out and be praised by others in a kingly majesty. I wanted to be someone everyone revered and loved for his brilliance. I still desire it even to this day, although my definition of "king" has changed as I grew older. Still, that day was essentially the day my life felt as if it had begun. From the morning to watching T.V. with my mother, it all felt like the start of something. Unknown to me at the time, it was the day my "king's journey" began. Finally, I was moving toward a dream I planned to make into reality. It was a dream that all started with a star and a crown.

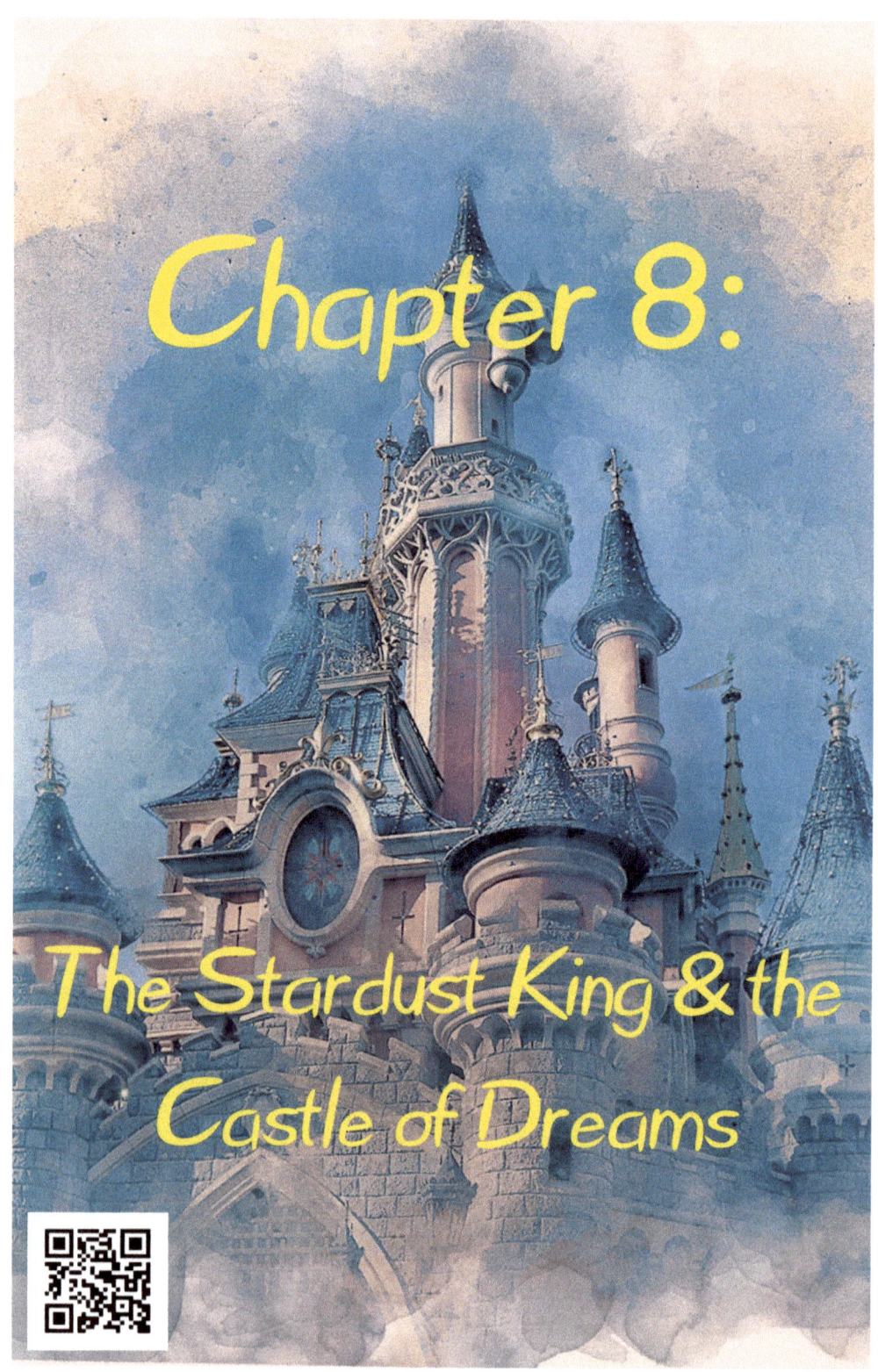

Chapter 8:

The Stardust King & the Castle of Dreams

CHAPTER VIII: The Stardust King & the Castle of Dreams

"Renewed shall be the blade that was broken. The crownless again shall be king."

- J.R.R. Tolkien

Simply put, there is no animal mightier than a lion. Lions are born royalty and respected amongst all, human and animal alike. Lions are both feared and revered for their power. The mere presence of a lion can invoke fear in the weakest of souls. Such is why lions are considered symbols for kings and queens throughout history. Such is why I consider lions to be the embodiment of my will. My name alone means "King," a burden I happily bear. Lions do not care for the opinions of others, nor do I.

STARDUST DREAMS

Whew! Quite the intense way to start the final chapter, right? I wanted to start this chapter off in a way that embodies my essence. My goal for the entire book was to be something uniquely unconventional. When I started this "authorship" career of mine, I was initially unsure of how to venture onto the path. Yet, with all great journeys, we must have the confidence to step forward. After all, that is how it all started on that fateful day. Readers of my first book should recall the event I am referencing. That is right – the day I wished to become king.

I was a young boy whenever I wished upon that lucky star. My wish was to become a King in my own right. But, I didn't know how I would do so or what it meant to become a king. Yet, I was determined to find out because that is what my heart was compelled to do. So, with my eyes on the sky and the heart in my stars, I began my lifelong journey to royalty.

STARDUST DREAMS

That fateful day will forever remain in my heart. Since then, I have always associated myself with stars in some capacity. Some people desire the moon; I desire the stars. For starters, stars are proof that there are other worlds aside from ours. The same star, which is billions of miles away, could be seen by two of the same people from different worlds.

It is truly a realization that life can exist outside of our galaxy. The same realization has always appealed to my heart. There is so much in this world I have yet to discover. Most of which I will never have time to discover fully. Knowing there are other worlds makes me want to discover those as well. Perhaps, in my next life, I will have that opportunity.

Maybe deep down, my wanderlust results from the "Kingly Spirit" in my heart. The sole ambition for wanting to discover and learn new things. Both of which to gain experience so I can fully grasp what it means to be a king. Although I don't understand what my version of being a king should be, I often analyzed others for specific blueprints. Over time, this allowed me to pick up on certain traits a king displays. One of the most important traits a king must have is ambition.

Being ambitious is by none the most important traits one must have in life. In my case, it is of the utmost importance to reach my goal of becoming a king. The reason why Julius Cesar was able to conquer Rome was due to ambition. The reason why Kobe Bryant became one of the greatest athletes ever was due to ambition. I have dubbed this ambition as a "kingly spirit." This is due to ambition being one of the main qualities a king must display. Moreso, those with a "kingly spirit" can often recognize others of the same.

In this regard, while rooted in ambition, I believe "kingly spirit" is unique to the individual. Anyone can display it, regardless of age, gender, race, nationality, etc. For example, "kingly spirit" can be exhibited by a child staying true to themselves. No matter how much the world tries to make the child change, they keep believing in themselves and their dreams. It is the will never to falter and continue forward on whichever path they choose. It is the lack of fear of being outcasted by others for staying true to one's ideals. All of which are rooted in an ever-burning ambition.

How do I know such to be true? Well, I was one of those children. There have been many times in my life when my spirit was tested. Admittedly, there have been many times when my spirit has cracked. However, it has never truly broken. There were so many times I wanted to give up. For those times, not because I wanted to, but because I felt the weight of the world. Yet every single time, I crawled out of whatever pit I found myself in. Getting back up every time we fall is a testament to one's persistence.

Persistence is a kingly trait rooted in ambition. The will to want something so badly, you will continue to pursue it, no matter the trials and tribulations. To overcome the world, you must be willing to fight for what you want. You must be the unstoppable force happily greeting the unmovable object, life. In my case, ambition and persistence have guided me to challenge the same world which tried to break me down. Every time I was ambitious and persistent, I was rewarded and punished.

Being ambitiously persistent is knowing you will fail more than you will succeed. Such is why the idea of persistence even exists. However, once you make it to the mountain you've been struggling to climb, you'll often come to a damning realization. You will realize there are always more steps to climb towards the top. The higher you climb, the harder it becomes to reach the top. Yet, we cannot be timid of the path before us. Instead, we must embrace it fully, knowing it will only be more challenging the higher we climb. In addition, we cannot be satisfied with mediocrity as it should never be a standard.

STARDUST DREAMS

No matter how long it takes, we cannot stop moving forward. Even if we need to crawl on our knees, we must keep onward towards our destiny. Such is the case with my now-defunct motto, "Walk Tall." Although I still do use it sometimes, it is not a phrase I live by wholeheartedly anymore. The main reason is because I've already fully embraced "Walk Tall" by realizing I've done so my entire life. The second is because "walk tall" began when my LSU journey did as well. Since my LSU saga has concluded, so has "walk tall."

Life is like a book; there's always a new chapter. There's no such thing as an ending, just a new beginning. I think that is what makes life all worth living. Not every chapter will be the best, but they'll be unique. The lessons we've learned along the way are essential as well. It is important to remember, however, one key aspect of life. There is no such thing as a painless lesson. My body is riddled with scars, bruises, bones that have never healed properly, etc.

STARDUST DREAMS

Every time I look at my old injuries, I realize how lucky I am to live through everything that tried to kill me. You see, scars are the body's natural tattoo. They're the stories to tell and the lessons we learned. I am a survivor, and every lesson that could've killed me didn't. I am thankful I survived and plan on doing so until I breathe my last breath. That is, not until I become the king I envision myself to be. Yet, even a king can take pride in his battle scars. If that is true, then so can I, the "self-proclaimed king."

"Self-proclaimed king" may be how others perceive me. To which I am completely fine with being seen as. As long as one can be happy with their reflection, then the image they see has true wealth. In this case, true royalty and prestige are in every definition of a monarch. Every time I look in a mirror, the image I see is a king. To the reader(s), I must offer a challenge. Every time you look into the mirror, make sure your crown isn't titled. You too, can become the king or queen of your own story.

STARDUST DREAMS

It all begins somewhere magical inside every person. It is a place where only you can go, nobody else. Be ambitious, persistent, and happy with who you are no matter what. It is easy to speak words of motivation but definitely much harder to take them to heart. It really is a lifestyle change most people do struggle with. Yet, it is proof your thoughts can determine your actions. As you think, so too shall you become. You shall come to bear the crown if you see yourself as royalty.

Above all else, if you have a dream, protect it with your life. You will spend every single day of your life alone in your head. Make that place a sanctuary only accessible by you. Make that same place something special and comforting. It should be a place you can retreat to when the world becomes too much to bear. Most importantly, let it be the gateway to your dreams as well. Allow that safe place to be similar to a vault. The most valuable item in that vault should be your dream(s).

STARDUST DREAMS

Do I have a place like this? Why yes, I most definitely do. It lies within my heart, and I visit it every day. In all honesty, I haven't done a spectacular job of keeping that place clean. Sometimes, things may "slip through the cracks" and create disorder. It's hard to prevent stuff from cluttering that safe space. In that regard, we have to realize there is always clutter to be removed. But, no matter how much clutter there may be, the vault that always protects my dreams shall remain undamaged.

Whew! That was quite the chapter to write if I say so myself. I don't know how this chapter will be perceived. Well, I am unsure how this entire book will be perceived. My first book received both praises and criticisms. Admittedly, I lost my motivation to cultivate another literary piece with the uproar I received.

It wasn't until realizing just how important my dreams are that I decided to dabble in writing once more. I know this book may create a similar or louder uproar. I know I will have difficulty promoting it as well. Nonetheless, my "kingly spirit" embraces these and any other challenges that may arise. Like a warrior gripping his sword and shield for battle, I am ready.

Now, allow me to re-introduce myself once more. My name is Arthur Calvin Price III. Son of Arthur Calvin Price Jr. and Joycelyn Denise Price and brother of Alex Joseph Price. I was the boy that wished upon a star. Now, I am the man working to make the wish come true. My dream is to become a king in my own right. I want to achieve something no person has before, nor will after that. I want to leave my mark on this world in a unique way. To accomplish such a feat, my dream is to become a king.

My story has become the real-life version of King Arthur's tale. That's right, I have already become a king in my own right. It took me a while to see it, but now I do. The throne is wherever I stand, not where I sit. My heart is the crown, although heavy, is one I proudly wear. I will continue to dream in my sanctuary, the castle of stardust.

To the reader(s), thank you for deciding to pick up this memoir. If you need me, you'll know where to find me. Just open this book up once more, that is. With that being said, until we meet again, my friends. Oh, what will I be doing till then? I'll be keeping my eyes on the sky and my heart in the stars. My dream of becoming a king began in the stars, remember? I certainly can't forget my dream – my stardust dream.

- FIN

STARDUST DREAMS

Thank you for reading "Stardust Dreams."

Please flip the page to view the ending artwork which is spread between two different pages. The piece is done by artist Alyssa Ochoa, 2022. I highly encourage you to please view it.

- Arthur C. Price III

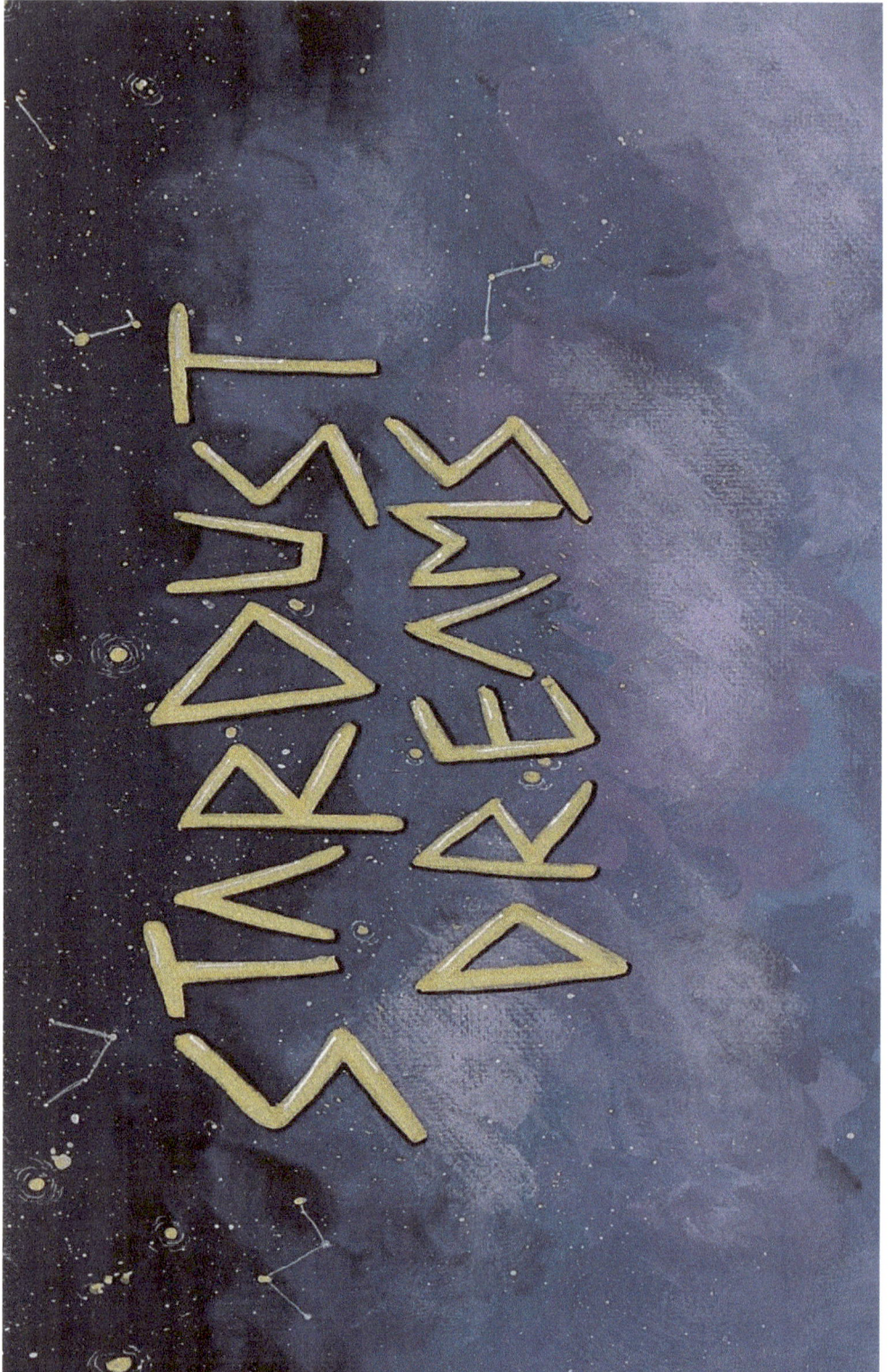

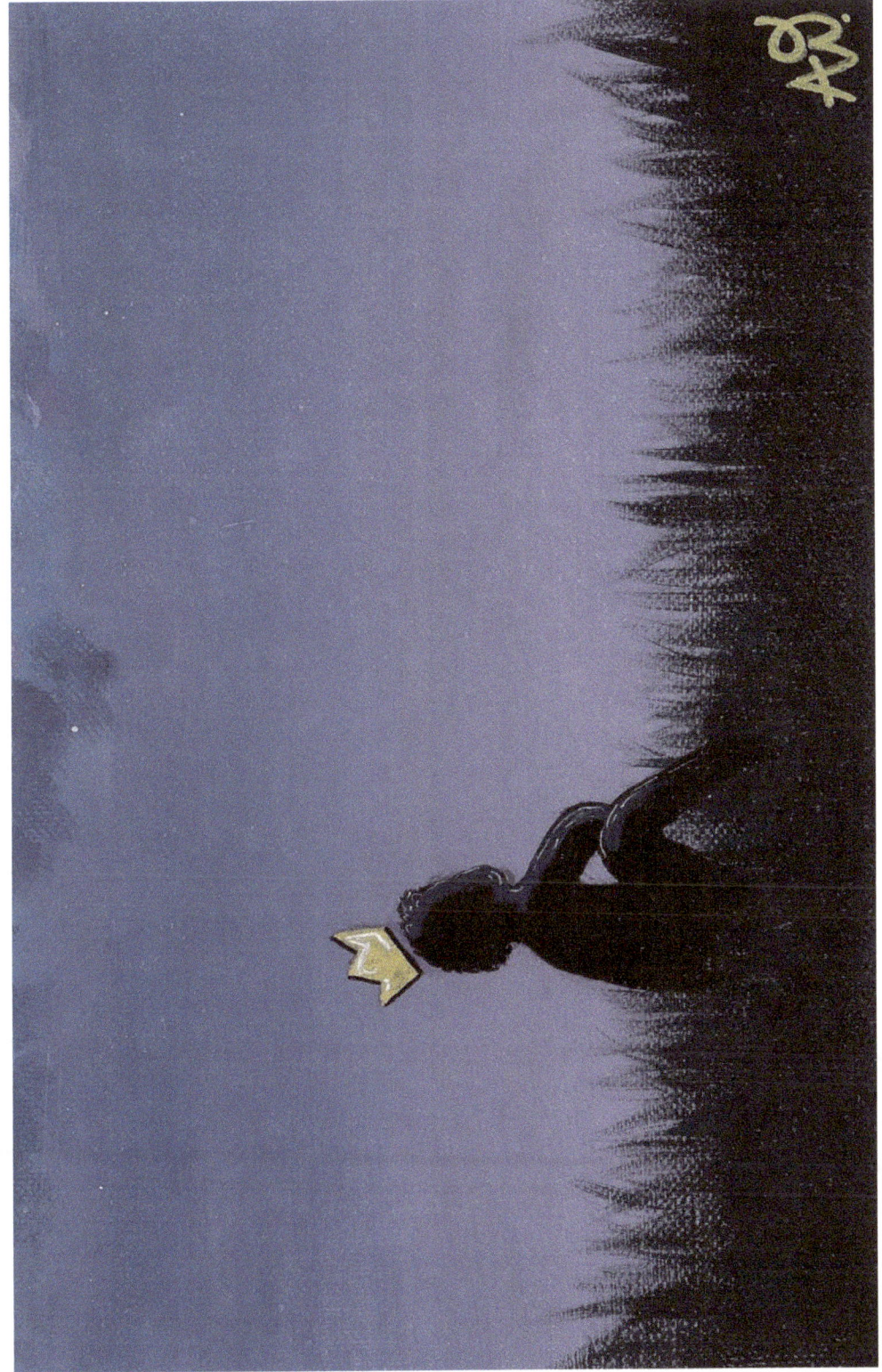

Photography Gallery

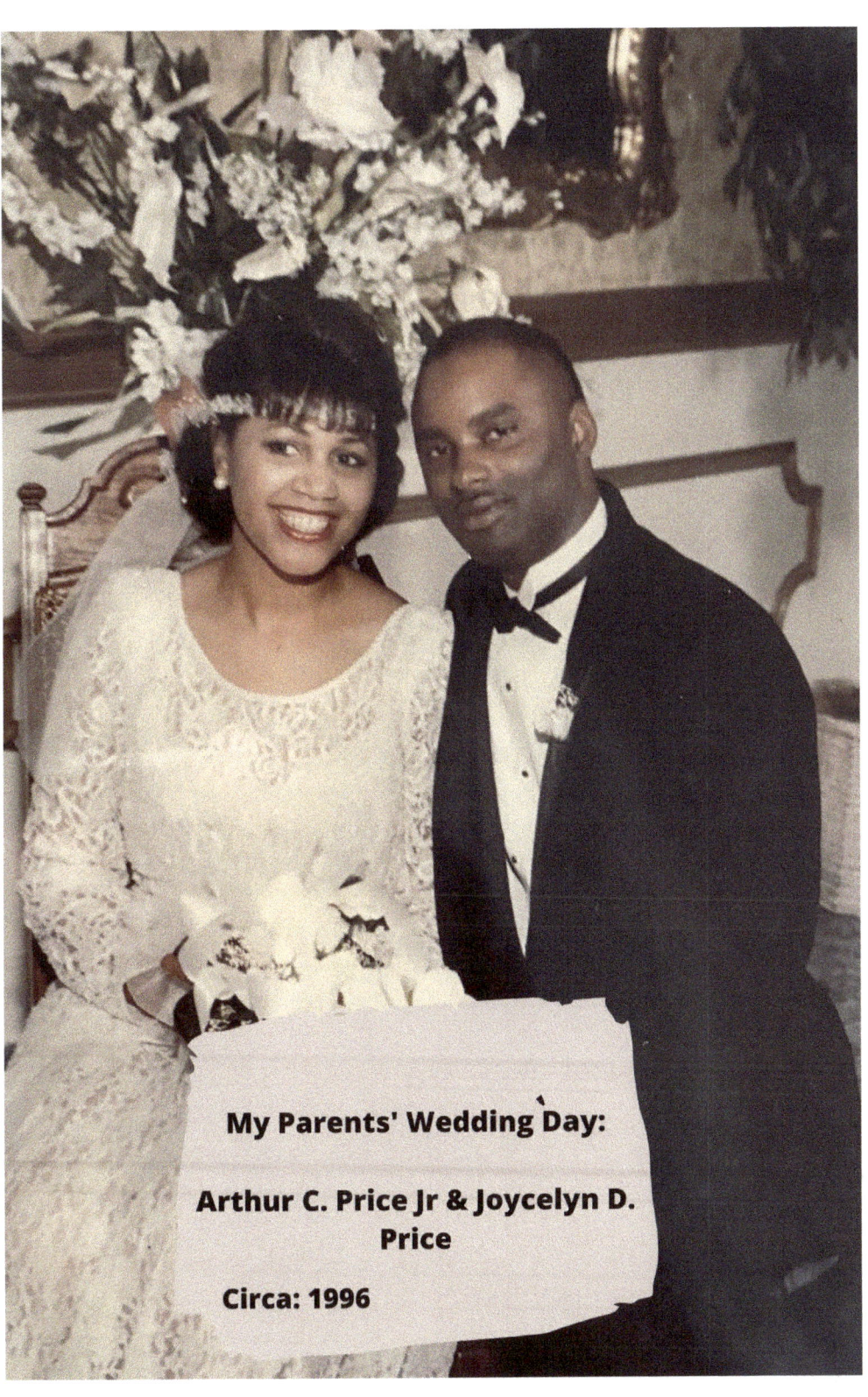

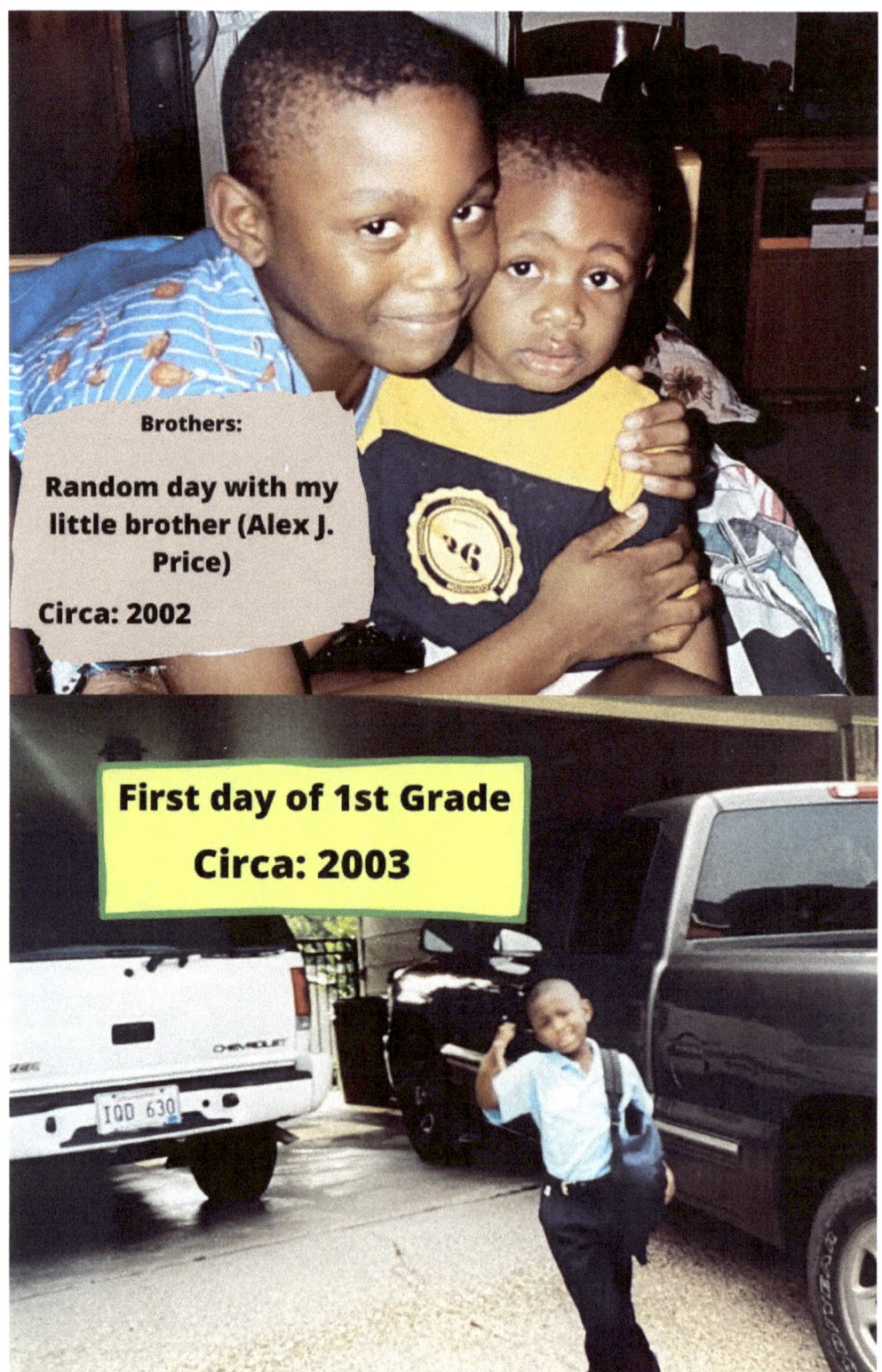

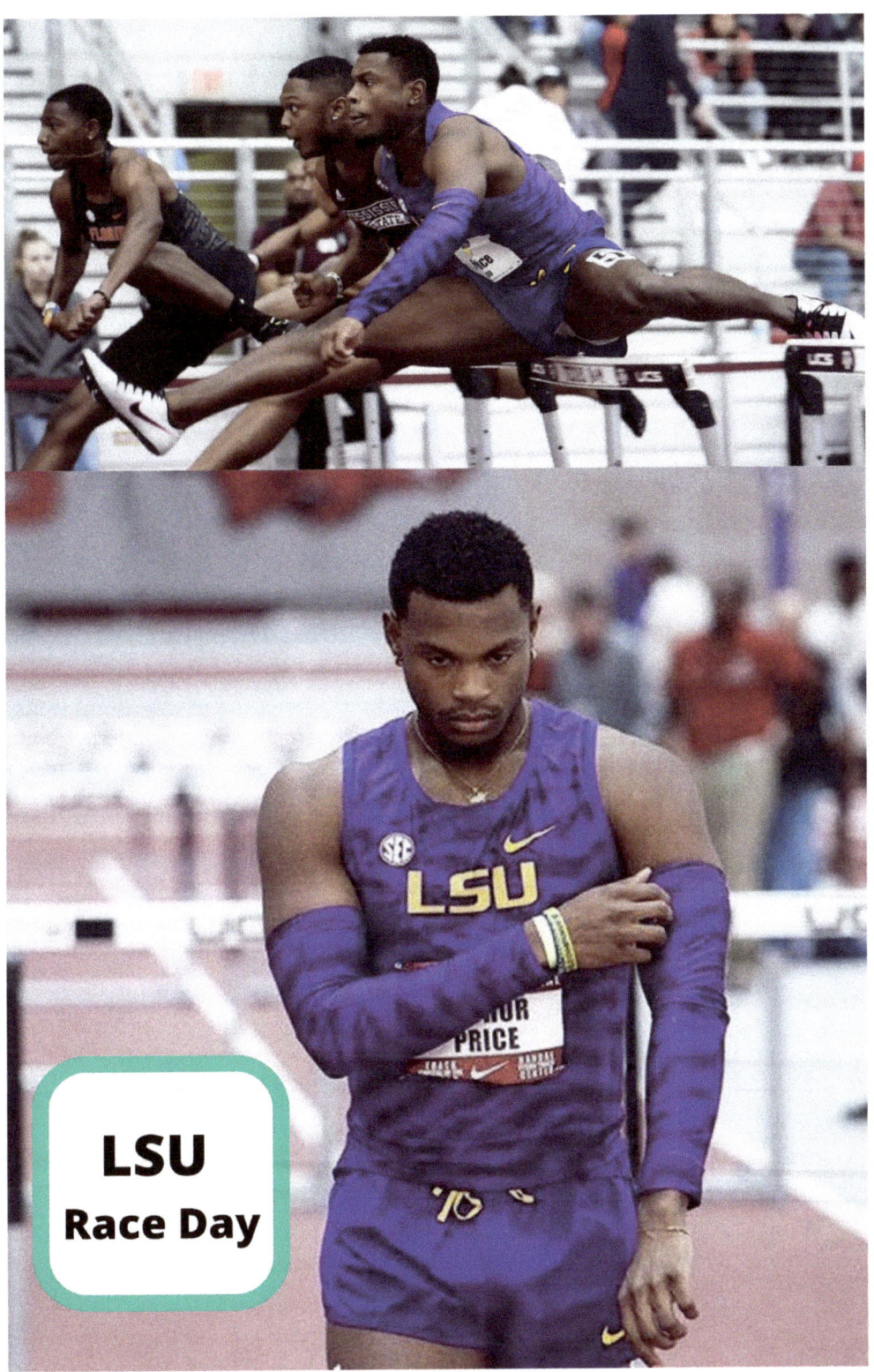

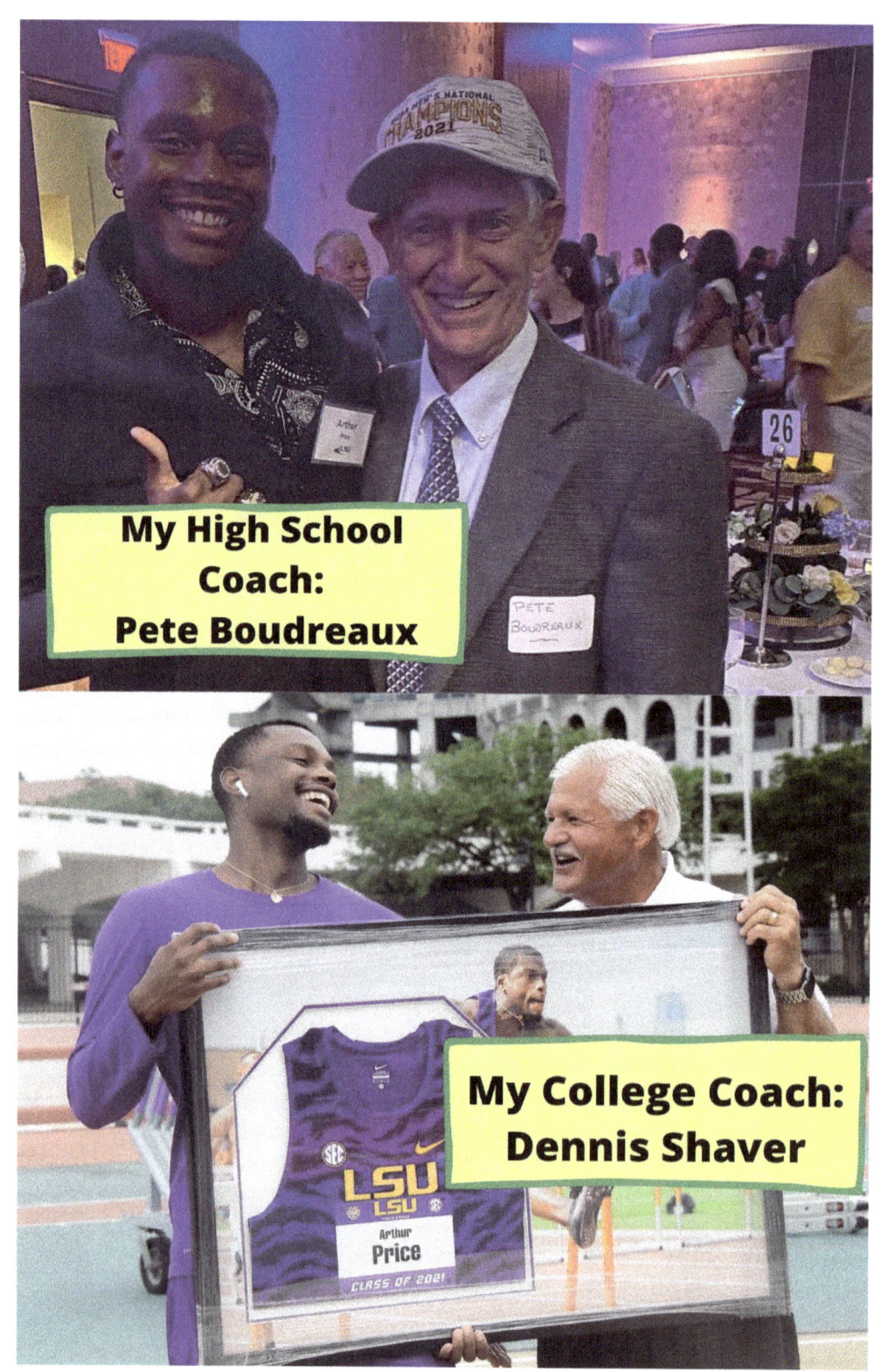

First Professional Race

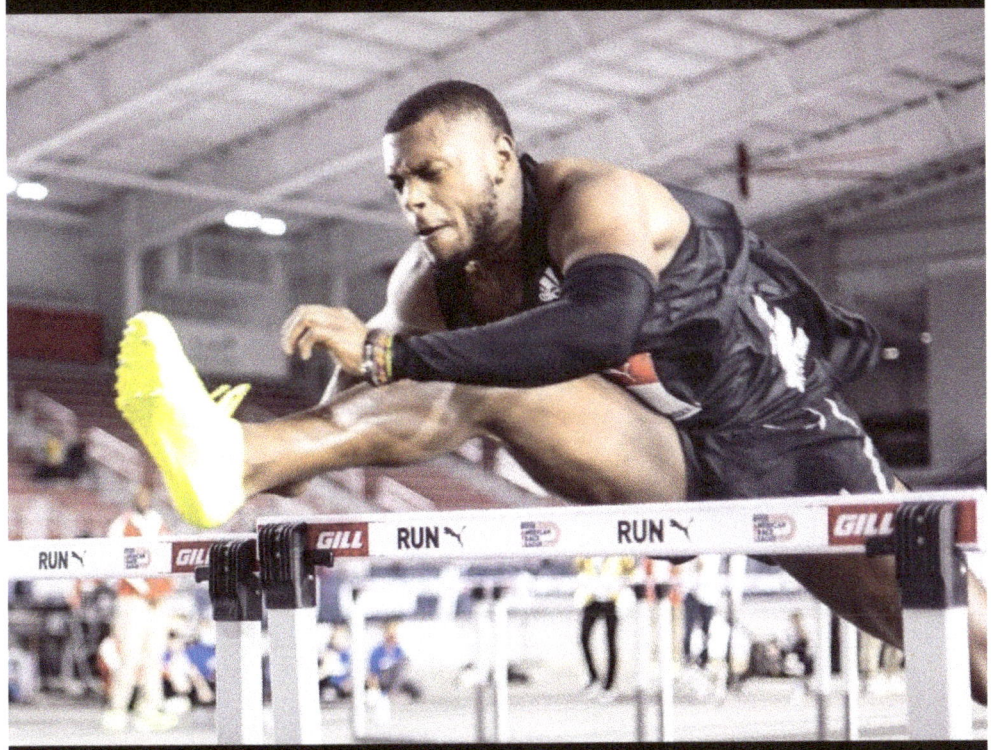

2022 Track & Field Season

STARDUST DREAMS
About the Author

Arthur C. Price III is an author from Baton Roue, Louisiana. His first published literary work, *"For the Man Who Walks Tall"* was published in October, 2020. In 2019, he received a bachelors degree in Psychology and Chemistry from LSU. As of 2021, he is a graduate student at Arizona State University. He is also a professional athlete who has garnered multiple achievements and notable awards.

His achievements include: Top 10 marks in LSU school history for two different events (110mH & 60mH), SEC (2019, 2021) & NCAA All-American (2019), 2020 Olympic Trials Qualifier, Ranked 8th in the USA and 96th in the world for the 110mH (2019). SEC Champion (LSU Team Title, 2019) and NCAA Champion (LSU Team Title, 2021).

Notable awards he has received are as follows: College of Humanities and Social Science Dean's List (2019), SEC Community Service Award (2020), LeJuan Simon Perseverance Award (2022).

To contact Arthur C. Price III, please utilize the respective resources listed below:

Website: www.arthurpriceiii.com

Social Media: @_arthurpriceiii (Instagram & Twitter)

Cell Phone #: 1-225-252-6508

Email Address: apric45@lsu.edu OR aprice8@asu.edu OR acp3@ymail.com

www.ingramcontent.com/pod-product-compliance
Lightning Source LLC
Chambersburg PA
CBHW051548010526
44118CB00022B/2618